T0140504

Indian Statistical Institute Series

The *Indian Statistical Institute Series* publishes high-quality content in the domain of mathematical sciences, bio-mathematics, financial mathematics, pure and applied mathematics, operations research, applied statistics and computer science and applications with primary focus on mathematics and statistics. Editorial board comprises of active researchers from major centres of Indian Statistical Institute. Launched at the 125th birth Anniversary of P.C. Mahalanobis, the series will publish high-quality content in the form of textbooks, monographs, lecture notes and contributed volumes. Literature in this series are peer-reviewed by global experts in their respective fields, and will appeal to a wide audience of students, researchers, educators, and professionals across mathematics, statistics and computer science disciplines.

More information about this series at http://www.springer.com/series/15910

Pranab Chakraborty · Subhamoy Maitra ·
Mridul Nandi · Suprita Talnikar

Contact Tracing
in Post-Covid World

A Cryptologic Approach

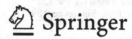
Springer

Pranab Chakraborty
Learning and Development
Wipro Limited
Bengaluru, Karnataka, India

Subhamoy Maitra
Applied Statistics Unit
Indian Statistical Institute
Kolkata, West Bengal, India

Mridul Nandi
Applied Statistics Unit
Indian Statistical Institute
Kolkata, West Bengal, India

Suprita Talnikar
Applied Statistics Unit
Indian Statistical Institute
Kolkata, West Bengal, India

ISSN 2523-3114   ISSN 2523-3122 (electronic)
Indian Statistical Institute Series
ISBN 978-981-15-9729-9   ISBN 978-981-15-9727-5 (eBook)
https://doi.org/10.1007/978-981-15-9727-5

Mathematics Subject Classification: 94A60, 68P25, 06E30, 94C10

This Springer imprint is published by the registered company Springer Nature Singapore Pte Ltd.
The registered company address is: 152 Beach Road, #21-01/04 Gateway East, Singapore 189721,
Singapore

To our colleagues in health sectors,
who are dedicating their lives to save us all.

Preface

We live in an age where exponential possibilities and shifting sands of uncertainties constantly redefine the "new normal". This time, it's COVID-19 that is controlling the playing field. Optimists will hope for a post-Covid world, while the rest, perhaps, will settle down to live with it for a long time, if not forever.

Given the pandemic nature of the infection and the high mortality rate associated with it, the world is facing an unprecedented challenge of tackling the disease at scale. On one hand, the people who are suffering from COVID-19 must have the best possible medical care and treatment, on the other hand, it is of utmost importance to ensure that the least number of uninfected people should come in close contact with the ones who are infectious. Moreover, an asymptomatic person may never know that he/she is infected (and possibly infectious), unless he/she is tested. At the same time, if it is known that a person is infected, then non-infected persons (other than the immediate family members and healthcare professionals) should be kept away from the infected person. It should be feasible to achieve this through the mobile phone network, software systems and tools and appropriate policies, processes and assumptions. The communication among the neighboring mobile phones can be achieved through the bluetooth protocol, while the location and other relevant information may be transmitted to some centralized authority through the mobile network.

Here, we assume that in the majority of circumstances, a person would choose to inform in case he/she is infected or in case he/she feels that he/she might have passed the infection to someone else. The other assumption is the trust of the community on the government and/or central administrative agencies so that the personally identifiable information of an individual (whether infected or not) does not get compromised or breached. It is known that the issue of individual privacy receives more attention in certain countries than in others. Thus, political and social issues may play a dominant role in deciding how an application related to "contact tracing" should be designed. From a practical point of view, manual contact tracing may still remain as one of the most effective options to limit the spread of the infection. However, with remarkable development in computation and communication, it is only natural that the world will eventually move towards digital systems to handle such a global pandemic.

In our point-of-view, cryptology will continue to be used as the fundamental science behind contact tracing software (applications/apps) given the security and privacy issues. In this book, we mostly concentrate on different contact tracing protocols from cryptologic (i.e., cryptographic and cryptanalytic) point of view. Such applications are being developed in many countries. The designers and developers come from government organizations, industries, academics, and research institutions. Given the nature of the outbreak of Covid-19, we observe knee-jerk reactions in most of the decision making processes. The same is true in the design of contact tracing protocols and their implementations. In a very short span covering only a couple of months, there are more than two dozens of proposals. At the same time, we read different critical reports in the media concerning the privacy issues. There are significant technical analyses as well in the form of research manuscripts. In that backdrop, we step in to write the first brief and comprehensive book in this domain, where we try to study the existing protocols, analyze them, and, finally, make a technical proposal for yet another logical design.

We start with an introductory chapter where we move from the informal discussions of contact-tracing proposals towards more technical analysis. We touch upon most of the existing digital contact tracing protocols and software that are being used and/or developed around the world. The transmission mechanism of the virus infection is discussed so that it can be understood how the contact tracing applications should be designed. Then we proceed towards the technical framework. The basic cryptologic primitives are explained briefly. This is needed to understand the security and privacy issues in digital contact tracing. With this, we enumerate a few well-known proposals and attempt to divide them into two categories: centralized and decentralized. From a cryptologic point of view, the design and analysis of decentralized contact tracing protocols carry more diverse and innovative ideas with better handling of privacy considerations.

We discuss some of the centralized applications in the second chapter, including Arogya Setu, TraceTogether, BlueTrace, OpenTrace, COVIDSafe, etc., that are currently in use in countries like India, Singapore or Australia. We study the elements and characteristics of these proposals from a cryptologic point of view. Next, we discuss the ROBERT protocol that has both the centralized and decentralized characteristics before concluding the chapter.

The third chapter analyzes the well-known decentralized applications such as DP3T and PACT. Such designs are available in the public domain for complete analysis. The technological giants like Apple and Google are also involved in similar efforts. Different cryptologic primitives and cryptanalytic issues need to be discussed in this perspective. We go through the design as well as design methodologies of these algorithms and also note the cryptanalytic results towards the evaluation of the protocols. A detailed comparison of such protocols is also discussed to highlight the advantages and disadvantages.

In the fourth and final chapter, we concentrate on how a digital contact tracing system should be designed maintaining the privacy of the users. We explain all the assumptions and cryptologic issues in this regard and present the exact problem statement to the best of our understanding. We specifically discuss higher order contact tracing in terms of the neighborhood of a neighborhood. This is in the direction that the people in the first neighborhood should be immediately tested, whereas the second layer should be quarantined. We present a detailed analysis of our generic proposal and then conclude. The book contains a detailed list of references at the end of each chapter.

The readers of this document should have some basic understanding of cryptology and security. At the same time, the first chapter of the book provides a brief background so that the materials can be followed to a large extent. Some basic ideas of computer and communication sciences might also be useful. This book is targeted towards students and researchers of any science and engineering discipline, and to engineers and professionals who work in the broad field of computation and communication.

At the same time, this material opens up some deep research problems for the experts who have a formal background on cryptology. The protocols that are analyzed and described here need to be studied carefully and cryptanalysis of certain aspects might be interesting research problems.

Before proceeding further, let us enumerate what is expected from this effort.

- This is the first comprehensive book on the design and analysis of contact tracing applications from a cryptologic viewpoint.
- This book provides a clear understanding of the design of contact tracing applications developed in different countries and continents.
- This brief document provides a link between very recent efforts related to digital contact tracing in COVID-19 scenario and a brief contextual literature review in this field.
- This draft presents a snapshot on how such applications are developed in a mobile distributed environment keeping in mind the issues of security and privacy, which is an important challenge in the domain of computer and communication sciences.
- This book is a short presentation of core concepts in the design and analysis of contact tracing applications.
- For experts in cryptology, this book points out possible research directions towards the security evaluation of existing contact tracing applications.

There are four listed authors of this book (in alphabetical order of surnames), but this effort is an outcome of the research efforts around the world. We thank all the researchers who are working in the domain of contact tracing. At the same time, we must acknowledge our family members and friends who constantly encouraged us in this trying time. Their kindness, love, and inspiration provided the prime motivation behind every word of this printed material. We also thank the support of Mr. Rishabh Kothary, a B.S. Mathematics and Scientific Computing student from

Indian Institute of Technology Kanpur, who worked as an intern during this effort and provided some interesting pointers. Dr. Dibyendu Roy, Dr. Pinakpani Pal, and Mr. Manmatha Roy of Indian Statistical Institute, Kolkata, have also contributed in providing additional inputs in this regard. We must acknowledge Mr. Shamim Ahmad, the Senior Editor from Springer Nature India Private Limited, for his able guidance. Last, but not the least, all the authors thank their respective family members for providing great support during this pandemic. Without all these encouragements and inputs, this book could not be written in a short time.

Each author likes to mention that all the views and recommendations expressed in this book (along with other co-authors) are entirely personal and not in any way related to each one's current organization. In addition, this work is purely based on a personal research interest and not related to their professional work.

The domain of digital contact tracing is an emerging field. However, we all wish that the present pandemic should be over as soon as possible. We will be happier than ever to have our world without any need of contact tracing, where this book would become useless. By any chance, are you still flipping the pages?

Bangalore, India   Pranab Chakraborty
Kolkata, India   Subhamoy Maitra
Kolkata, India   Mridul Nandi
July 2020   Suprita Talnikar

Contents

About the Authors

Pranab Chakraborty is Senior Manager at the Learning and Development team of Wipro Limited, Bengaluru, India. He earned his graduate degree in computer science from the Indian Statistical Institute, Kolkata, India, and undergraduate degree in electronics and telecommunications engineering from Jadavpur University, Kolkata, India. He has implemented various network protocol stacks including TCP/IP and played different organizational roles including that of a technical architect and technical delivery manager apart from his current involvement in the behavioral and leadership development field. He has a special interest in the research areas of cryptology.

Subhamoy Maitra is Senior Professor at the Applied Statistics Unit of the Indian Statistical Institute, Kolkata, India. He earned his Ph.D. and graduate degree in computer science from the Indian Statistical Institute, Kolkata, India, and undergraduate degree in electronics and telecommunications engineering from Jadavpur University, Kolkata, India. Post working in the domain of hardware and software engineering for a few years, Prof. Maitra joined the Indian Statistical Institute, Kolkata, as a faculty in 1997. Having around 6000 citations to his name, Prof. Maitra has authored several books and around 200 research papers in the area of cryptology and quantum information.

Mridul Nandi is Professor at the Applied Statistics Unit of the Indian Statistical Institute, Kolkata, India. Earlier, he worked for the National Institute of Standards and Technology (NIST), USA, as one of the technical members in the selection process of the SHA3 hash function. His research areas focus on different aspects of cryptography, including hash functions, MAC, authenticated encryption, identity (or attribute) based encryption, IoT, hardware implementation and lightweight cryptography. He is the co-designer of COLM (authenticated encryption), selected as a winner in the security category of CAESAR portfolio. Algorithms of his designed 10 lightweight ciphers were selected for the second round of NIST lightweight standard process. He actively publishes papers in top tier conferences like Eurocrypt, Crypto, Asiacrypt, FSE and renowned journals.

Suprita Talnikar is Senior Research Fellow at the Applied Statistics Unit of the Indian Statistical Institute, Kolkata, India. She is pursuing her Ph.D. in Computer Science, under the supervision of Prof. Mridul Nandi. She completed her M.Sc. in Mathematics from Visvesvaraya National Institute of Technology, Nagpur, India, with a gold medal, and her B.Sc. in Physics, Computer Science and Mathematics from Rashtrasant Tukadoji Maharaj Nagpur University, Nagpur, India. Her research focuses on various areas of cryptography, with particular interest in provable security and cryptanalysis in symmetric key cryptography.

Chapter 1
Introduction and Preliminaries

Abstract In this chapter, we will discuss the basic understanding of contact tracing software and the related cryptographic techniques. The underlying models of computation and communication will be explained. A standard smartphone can be considered as the basic device and there will be communication among those devices using Bluetooth technology. The data transfer between the mobile device and the backend server (might be controlled by governmental authorities) will be taken care of by the standard data communication channel provided by the service provider. Social issues related to privacy will also be touched upon in this introductory chapter.

1.1 Introduction

Consider the design of an application such that if you come locationally close to one of your friends then your mobile phone will give you a signal. There could be two different approaches to implementation. In one approach, the location of the phones could be continuously analyzed by some location tracking system. Whenever the system finds two phones in close proximity of each other, it would check whether one phone number is in the contact list of the other. If found, then both the phones will be notified with some characteristic sound, vibration, or a message. What are the problems in this approach?

1. First of all, in a location, there are a large number of mobile phones and therefore such a matching algorithm would possibly have huge costs associated with computation and communication.
2. The complexity of the algorithm would get compounded due to the dynamic and real-time nature of the process.
3. In addition to the computational issues, there is a serious privacy concern. If the application is running in a central server, the server would have the location histories of everyone using such an application.

BLUETOOTH- BASED SOLUTION. There is another clever option that may not need to depend upon any location tracking systems. In this option, the communication happens through the Bluetooth technology. Hence, the two devices can communicate with each other only when the friends who own the two devices come in close proximity to each other, say, for example, within a distance of 10 m. Since in this approach the phones would use the Bluetooth technology, the devices would not have to depend upon the mobile network services. This is exactly the approach of Bluetooth-based [49] automated contact tracing [32, 34] solutions. If a person is diagnosed SARS-CoV-2 positive, then the people around him/her can be informed about their risk of getting infected as long as all of them have the contact tracing app running on their mobile phones. The protocols that are used in such Bluetooth-based notification systems are referred to as digital contact tracing protocols. Implementing such a system is rather straightforward given the maturity of Bluetooth technology. That is why in the present scenario, many countries and certain private entities have planned to launch such a system on priority. In some of the countries, such systems have already been rolled out. Given the level of urgency due to the ongoing pandemic, and the severe competitive and volatile business environment, the possibility of standardization of such software systems around the world seems elusive. Also, some of the privacy and security issues could be country-specific. Under this scenario, our main motivation is to explain the algorithms of contact tracing protocols, identify the cryptographic primitives used, and analyze the security and architecture of these systems. We present our analysis of the apps and protocols that are already being used in Singapore, Australia, the USA, India, and some of the European countries. Technological giants Google and Apple together have come up with a set of APIs [4] for exposure notification and several researchers across the world have proposed a formidable range of sophisticated cryptographic protocols and frameworks. It is understood that for travel and for many other purposes, some kind of passports related to SARS-CoV-2 could become essential [36] in the coming days. For example, the Government of India has proposed integration of e-pass functionality, which is meant for any interstate travel during the restricted movement phase, within the Aarogya Setu contact tracing app. Users of the app may also be allowed to apply and get approval for the e-passes through Aarogya Setu app's user interface.

1.2   Background

Before we understand or analyze the digital contact tracing systems, let us delve deep into the question of "why is contact tracing needed."

First, contact tracing is a tool that primarily helps health agencies and state health departments to predict and control the growth trajectory of an infectious disease. The use of such a tool is essential in an outbreak, epidemic, or pandemic situation.[1]

---

[1]Due to the epidemic spread of SARS-CoV-2, the WHO (World Health Organization) has declared it a pandemic in March 2020.

However, not all infectious diseases can be tracked using contact tracing. For example, dengue is transmitted by mosquitoes that act as carriers of the virus and any contact tracing effort for dengue would involve tracking the movement of infectious mosquitoes—which can be an exciting topic for a sci-fi movie but no agency or state health department would be dreaming of doing that at this point of time. So when we talk of contact tracing, we are talking about contagious diseases that can be transmitted from human to human directly or via a passive surface like fomites (i.e., objects or materials that are likely to carry infection, such as clothes, utensils, and furniture). So, digital contact tracing solutions (along with the manual tracing) based on mobile applications could efficiently achieve epidemic control on a large scale.

Second, contact tracing also helps the epidemiologists to study the transmission mechanism of a contagious disease. Usually, for a new disease like SARS-CoV-2, epidemiologists may refine the standard parameters of the system dynamic models (like SIR or SEIR) [54] based on the stages through which the disease evolves while the contagion may go through certain mutations. These models help in predicting the way the number of people within a geographical region, under the epidemiological compartments, like Suspected (S), Exposed (E), Infectious (I), Recovered (R), etc., may vary with time.

Finally, and most importantly, contact tracing can help the general public in many ways. Those who might have come in contact with an infected individual(s) get to know of the exposure events and therefore their risks of infection through this process. In such cases, the health agencies also provide prophylactic and/or preventive care for such individuals. They are monitored on a daily basis for any development of the symptoms. Also, in case there is a need to quarantine infected or exposed (i.e., at risk) individuals, the health agencies and administration provide such measures based on the findings of the contact tracing process.

Thus, there arises the need for a contact tracing mechanism that does this job as precisely and swiftly as possible.

1.2.1 Did Contact Tracing Help in the Past?

Indeed, there are a number of instances where contact tracing has helped in effectively controlling and limiting the spread of some diseases. For example, [17] smallpox was eradicated by contact tracing and not by universal immunization. In the case of Ebola, it has been successfully used for many years. A CDC (Center for Disease Control and Prevention) report [25] on 2014 Ebola outbreak response highlights that

> contact tracing is a key part of the outbreak ...it's been used in each of the previous 20 Ebola outbreaks over the past 40 years to successfully control Ebola.

Another recent article [31] by two physicians Hart and Yarwood, mentions how contact tracing has helped to limit the spread in case of HIV and meningitis infections.

They consider contact tracing and isolation of infected or at-risk individuals as two important assets that may help in limiting the spread of SARS-CoV-2.

1.2.2 How Is Contact Tracing Done Manually?

The manual contact tracing process starts by identifying the initial set of infected individuals (called the *index cases*) who have been tested positive to the contagion under study and then interviewing each such individual to find out the possible *close contacts*, who might have contracted the infection while coming in close proximity with an *index case*. There is no strict definition of *close contact* or *close proximity*. We can borrow the definition [31] given by Queensland Health as per the guidelines of Communicable Disease Network, Australia that says

> Close contacts are those who have had face-to-face contact with a confirmed case for a period more than 15 minutes, or those who have shared an enclosed space with a confirmed case for more than two hours.

A comparable definition comes from United State's Center for Disease Control and Prevention which states in their website [18] that

> For SARS-CoV-2, a close contact is defined as any individual who was within 6 feet of an infected person for at least 15 minutes starting from 2 days before illness onset (or, for asymptomatic patients, 2 days prior to positive specimen collection) until the time the patient is isolated.

However, there are observed incidents that contradict the above-mentioned understanding that it takes 15 min or more for the infection to get transmitted. For example, it has been reported [5] by a group of virologists that confirmed transmission took place between two asymptomatic individuals who came near each other for a brief period of time in the company cafeteria where one person passed a saltshaker to another.

In the manual contact tracing process, the contacts are monitored for an *incubation period* to see if any of them develop symptoms and eventually test positive, in which case he/she is isolated, treated and in turn interviewed to identify his/her close contacts or in case any of them does not show any symptom (or test negative), that person is declared to be not at risk. From an algorithmic point of view, this entire process is repeated for each index case. These data points of primary, secondary, or tertiary contacts starting with the index cases can also be used for analyzing the transmission dynamics, infection clusters, and different types of searches.

1.2.3 Challenges and Issues of Manual Contact Tracing

We briefly mention some challenges and issues which are to be faced in a manual contact tracing process.

1. The main challenge of manual contact tracing is that it is a painstaking process and at the same time resource intensive. It takes time and effort to do a detailed interview of an infected individual and still, it remains error-prone since it depends on how well the infected individual may remember the necessary information like the route map (places where he/she went in the last 14 days, in case of SARS-CoV-2) and the people who came in close contact with him/her in that route.
2. Privacy and confidentiality: Every individual has a right to the confidentiality of his/her medical condition. Hence, at the time of alerting an individual about the possible exposure that might have happened, the health practitioner is not expected to disclose the identity of the infected individual(s).
3. Ethics and legalities: The health agency or department has an ethical and (in most countries) legal obligation to share the information about the risk factor to the individuals who might have contracted the contagion from some other infectious individual.
4. Social stigma: Sometimes, the contacts may feel discouraged to share all information in the fear of stigma, discrimination, abuse, or even ostracization within the society.

1.2.4 The Transmission Mechanism

For analyzing digital contact tracing systems, it is useful to have some knowledge of the transmission mechanism of the SARS-CoV-2 virus. We present here a brief summary of our current understanding. Since SARS-CoV-2 is a newly discovered virus, the understanding about the mechanism of its transmission is expected to evolve over a period of time. As per the current understanding [58] of the World Health Organization (WHO), the virus can get transmitted from symptomatic and pre-symptomatic individuals to others who have come in direct or close contact with the infected individuals. Additionally, the transmission can happen through a passive surface that retains active virus landing on it in the form of respiratory droplets from symptomatic, pre-symptomatic or asymptomatic individuals. The shedding of the virus from the respiratory tract of symptomatic individuals appears to be highest in the first 3 days from the onset of the symptom. On average, a pre-symptomatic individual starts showing symptoms of SARS-CoV-2 after 5–6 days and in some cases as late as 14 days. A pre-symptomatic person may test positive to SARS-CoV-2, 1–3 days before the symptoms of the disease appear. The maximum amount of confusion lies in the case of asymptomatic individuals. In one of the latest updates [60], WHO has mentioned the following:

> A subset of studies and data shared by some countries on detailed cluster investigations and contact tracing activities have reported that asymptomatically infected individuals are much less likely to transmit the virus than those who develop symptoms.

In summary, the following points are so far known about the transmission mechanism:

- The chance of transmission is highest from symptomatic individuals in the first 3 days after the onset of the symptom.
- Symptomatic individuals remain infectious throughout the duration of disease in his/her body.
- Some pre-symptomatic individuals may be infectious on an average 5–6 days or in the worst case 14 days before the symptoms start showing.
- The transmission can also happen through passive surfaces [59] and the virus may remain active on such surfaces for a few hours and up to several days.
- Asymptomatically infected individuals are much less likely to transmit the virus as compared to symptomatic or pre-symptomatic individuals.
- There is also one more category, called *oligosymptomatic transmission* that has been mentioned in certain research publications (e.g., in [55]), which indicates that for some individuals the symptoms are so mild that they may even be misinterpreted as asymptomatic cases.

We should also remember that the nature or behavior of the virus may change over time. By analyzing virus genomes from several infected persons with SARS-CoV-2, researchers have reportedly [41] identified close to 200 recurrent genetic mutations in the virus. This reflects how it may be adapting and evolving to its human hosts.

1.3   Digital Contact Tracing Systems

Although, in the last few years researchers have conceived contact tracing systems via mobile phones (e.g., the published work of Farrahi et al. [27], the research published by Zhang et al. [62] and, that of Altuwaiyan et al. [3]), there was no significant implementation or experimentation done on digital contact tracing systems in any country prior to the SARS-CoV-2 outbreak. In the last few months, top researchers, organizations, and governments across the world have started proposing a number of competing protocols, frameworks, API systems, and apps. Many of these proposals have also envisaged the possibility of how various systems may be used across multiple countries or geographical regions. However, so far, none of the proposals has considered the co-existence and interoperability of multiple solutions and systems. We briefly touched upon this in Chap. 4.

The primary driving factor behind the digital contact tracing systems is the usage of cutting edge technology to efficiently scale up a time-tested epidemiological method and thereby stop, control or at least reduce the break-neck speed with which SARS-CoV-2 is spreading across the globe and creating havoc in our lives. The central idea is to use an automated method of detecting contact events of two mobile phones coming in proximity with each other and acting as a proxy to the event of two individuals coming in close contact.

1.3.1 Challenges and Issues of Digital Contact Tracing

While the digital contact tracing systems can circumvent the main challenge of manual contact tracing systems of being painstaking and resource intensive, it faces some imminent new challenges as follows.

- What would happen to those individuals who do not have his/her own mobile device?
- Will the digital system support the feature phones or would it be only implemented for smartphones?
- How reliable and accurate will be such alert systems?
- What happens if a significant part of the population does not install and/or enable the system in their devices due to some reason (e.g., suboptimal customer experience)?

Other related issues that are applicable in manual contact tracing systems may continue to impact the digital version as well, like

- privacy and confidentiality,
- ethical and legal issues, and
- social stigma,

as discussed earlier. Thus, an important question is

> Will digital contact tracing systems replace the manual contact tracing process?

A short answer to this question is *no*. With a little more elaboration, we can say that digital contact tracing systems may not replace the manual process completely at least in the short term. To understand the reasons, let us look at what WHO has mentioned as the three basic steps of contact tracing (we copy the whole text from [57] in the following three points).

- Contact identification: Once someone is confirmed as infected with a virus, contacts are identified by asking about the person's activities and the activities and roles of the people around them since the onset of illness. Contacts can be anyone who has been in contact with an infected person: family members, work colleagues, friends, or healthcare providers.
- Contact listing: All persons considered to have contact with the infected person should be listed as contacts. Efforts should be made to identify every listed contact and to inform them of their contact status, what it means, the actions that will follow, and the importance of receiving early care if they develop symptoms. Contacts should also be provided with information about the prevention of the disease. In some cases, quarantine or isolation is required for high-risk contacts, either at home or in hospital.
- Contact follow-up: Regular follow-up should be conducted with all contacts to monitor for symptoms and test for signs of infection.

Once a health agency confirms that an individual (say *B*) is infected, it should immediately initiate the process of identifying the close contacts by interviewing *B* and not wait for the apps installed in the mobile devices of those individuals to raise the alarm. Not only would it be a waste of precious time, but there is also a possibility that some of those close contacts (e.g., kids or aged relatives) may not carry separate smartphones. Additionally, in many developing or under-developed countries, the number of mobile devices per family (especially in rural areas) can be limited in number. In majority of those cases, mobile devices may just be feature phones instead of smartphones.

Hence, towards following the basic steps of contact identification, contact listing, and contact follow-up for the contacts who can immediately be identified by the infected person, manual process of contact tracing may remain the most efficient as well as the most effective approach. Another important factor is digital contact tracing systems in most of the countries would be introduced as a choice and not as a mandate. So every individual can voluntarily opt-in or decide to opt-out. The absolute number of people who prefer to opt-out can be significant even under a wide-spread adoption of digital contact tracing apps. In fact, an individual who decides to opt-out may have an expectation that state health agencies would pro-actively reach out to them in case it is found out that he/she came in contact with *B*.

1.3.1.1 Did *B* Infect *A* or Was It the Other Way Around?

Let us now briefly revisit the case of *A* and *B* where *A* comes in close contact with *B* and a few days later *B* shows symptoms and tests positive to SARS-CoV-2. At this point, *A* is expected to be alerted through the manual or digital contact tracing process that she may also watch out for possible symptoms and if required test herself (for SARS-CoV-2). At this point, it may appear natural to assume that *A* has contracted the virus from *B*, but based on the analysis of the previous section we can logically deduce that it could as well be the other way round. For example, the situation might have been that—*A* (a pre-symptomatic but infected individual) has come in close contact with *B* (not infected at that point of time) and transmitted the virus during that contact. *B*'s symptoms have appeared earlier than *A* and that is why it may incorrectly be concluded that *B* has infected *A*. There are instances in the documentation of some contact tracing systems where this incorrect conclusion has been drawn and hence while using such systems in the future, users may be alerted with incomplete or incorrect information (of course unintentionally).

1.4 The Technical Framework

Necessity is the mother of all inventions and humanity's desire of getting rid of the current crisis created by the worldwide pandemic, is the mother of all necessities. Hence, the research, technical, and professional communities from various fields across the world are joining hands together to conceptualize, design, and implement the digital contact tracing systems at a rapid pace. Due to the involvement of renowned experts (especially from the cryptologic community), many of these systems include innovative protocols and security designs. At the same time due to the rapid pace, some design features appear to be less secure, error-prone, or contrary to their design goals. Over a period of time, we believe these inaccuracies will be taken care of. In the next two chapters (Chaps. 2 and 3), we analyze the pros and cons of various designs by comparing these proposals against their intended objectives and goals. Finally, in Chap. 4, we will present a generic proposal and aim to predict the future course of digital contact tracing systems and the evolving role of cryptology. The motivation of our proposal is to outline how a design could be attempted by balancing different types of (and sometimes contradicting) requirements.

Any innovation happens at the intersection of three factors:

- desirability,
- viability, and
- feasibility.

We have already discussed at length the need for digital contact tracing systems—the desirability factor is therefore addressed. Viability does not appear to be a challenge for this system as every Government and the Ministry of Health of every country is talking about its urgent need and would eventually promote and champion the usage of such systems. So what remains is to explore the factor of technical feasibility.

1.4.1 Technical Feasibility

The number of smartphone users and the number of mobile phone users in the world are estimated to be 3.5 billion and 4.8 billion respectively. Hence, there are about 3 billion people who do not carry any type of mobile phone. The implication of this is as follows.

- There is no technology at this point that can enable digital contact tracing system (DCTS) for everybody in the world. However, in many developed countries, the number of people using smartphones can be quite high, and hence in such countries, a successful roll-out of DCTS may prove to be extremely effective in controlling the spread of the disease. For example, in Singapore, smartphone penetration is estimated [37] to be around 78%.
- Smartphone app-based digital contact tracing systems can be implemented quickly to achieve most of the objectives of contact tracing as outlined by WHO.
- Feature phone-based systems would have technical limitations and can't be as seamless as app-based systems. However, it is possible to envisage such systems.
- Realistically, Governments and Health Departments have to judiciously use a hybrid of manual and digital contact tracing systems to get the best possible outcome in the current situation.

- Feasibility of detecting transmission through passive surfaces can and must be explored after doing rapid prototyping and experimentation.

1.4.2 System Goals and Objectives

There can be some broad level system goals for such a system, including but not limited to-

- Achieving contact tracing objectives as per guidelines from WHO,
- Prompt notification of alert,
- Epidemiological analysis, prediction, and control,
- Robustness, reliability, and endurance,
- Precision and accuracy,
- System integrity,
- Confidentiality, security, and privacy,
- Interoperability (across regions or across device types or across implementation systems),
- Extensibility,
- Re-usability (in future scenarios), and
- Upward compatibility.

At present, some of the proposals are touching upon many of these goals. However, none of the proposals comprehensively addresses all of these. This is quite natural given the short span and urgency of the designs. It would be desirable that in the near future every system explicitly states their exact positions with respect to all these goals.

In almost all the systems, explicit focus has been given to privacy and security goals because, in many countries, the law is quite strict with respect to confidentiality, security, and privacy.

1.4.3 System Architecture: Options and Trade-Offs

The basic use case involves two individuals (*A* and *B*) and their mobile devices (say A and B respectively) acting as their proxies. When the two individuals come in close contact with each other the system must ensure that A records the presence of B and vice versa. From a theoretical perspective, it could be possible to envisage a system where it is sufficient to have only one device (say A) recording the presence of the other device (here B). However, none of the launched or proposed systems falls in this category—hence we would not analyze such solutions. At this point of time, there is a general agreement in the technical and research community that the most suitable option to achieve this functionality is to use the Bluetooth Low Energy (BLE) protocol [14]. BLE, earlier referred as Bluetooth Smart, is a wireless personal area network technology [12, 14], that has been designed and marketed by Bluetooth

Special Interest Group (SIG) for creating applications around fitness, smart homes, security, proximity, etc. It is different from the classic Bluetooth Basic Rate/Enhanced Data Rate (BR/EDR) protocol but both use the same 2.4 GHz frequency range and can co-exist in the same device. A variety of mobile platforms (iOS, Android, etc.) and generic operating systems (macOS, Windows 10, etc.) provide native support for BLE. BLE protocol [50] can operate in two different topologies—broadcast topology and connection topology. In broadcast topology, devices may advertise packets (as broadcaster) with a payload of 31 bytes to other devices that are repeatedly scanning (as receivers) to receive advertised packets in a non-connectable mode. There are no inherent provisions of security or privacy in broadcast topology and it is a fast and easy to use the technique for a device to send a short packet to a number of peers simultaneously. In case a device needs to send a payload larger than 31 bytes, there is a provision to use scan response technique to send an additional 31-byte secondary payload in broadcast topology. A device may periodically alternate between the broadcaster role and the receiver role. In the connection topology mode, devices can communicate bidirectionally by establishing a connection between a device playing the role of a central (master) and the other playing the role of a peripheral (slave). A device can act as a central and peripheral at the same time where one central may connect to one more peripheral and similarly a peripheral may connect to a number of centrals. In connection topology mode, devices can have a finer grained control on the data being shared and hence is more secure than the broadcast topology mode. The BLE specification ensures interoperability among multiple device types through two profiles—Generic Access Profile (GAP) and Generic Attribute Profile (GATT) that act as the entry points of the higher layer APIs to the BLE protocol stack.

ASSUMPTIONS. Devices using BLE let the other devices know about its presence by broadcasting discovery packets (in certain intervals through one of the approved channels) and scanning/recording the broadcast packets received from the other devices. The intent is to use the information contained in the packets to detect at a later point of time whether A (mobile device of A) came in close proximity to B (mobile device of B who eventually got tested as SARS-CoV-2 positive) for a duration that is sufficiently long to transmit the virus from one to the other (it can be either B to A or A to B) assuming one of them was not infected at the time when they met. In this scenario, the assumptions are as follows.

- Both the devices A and B were switched on with Bluetooth enabled or Bluetooth scanning enabled (and in some situations, there is an additional constraint of using the app in the foreground mode).
- Each of the devices has the same app installed. In each device, the app takes care of broadcasting and recording the discovery packets sent and received via BLE interface.
- The BLE protocol correctly captures the *close proximity* situation and devices do not capture packets from other devices that are either too far off or have stayed close only for a brief period of time. Here, we must highlight that certain aspects would not be detectable like, whether A and B were wearing masks at the time

when they met or whether an infected person was present some time back and touched a surface through which A or B might have got exposed to the contagion.

Central Server. Since the detection of the event that "B is positive" happens at a point of time much later than when A and B met, the question comes as to how device A would come to know of it. It is unlikely that at the point of time when this information becomes known, A would be in close range of B—hence alerting mechanism can't be built using BLE. If somehow B stores the phone number of A (or at least one of the phone numbers in case of dual-SIM phones), B may be able to intimate A. However, that might not be appropriate from the security and privacy perspective. Ideally, B should not learn any extra information (like identity, phone number, IMEI number, etc.) about A or her phone, other than storing some packet values from A. The same expectation holds for packets received by A from B. Hence, to solve this deadlock, we may introduce a (trusted or semi-trusted) third entity (called C as the server that includes a database) which would facilitate the process that leads to alerting A about the fact that she came in close contact with an infected individual B some days back and hence she must consult a health professional to seek guidance or get checked.

TYPES OF DATA COMMUNICATION IN MEETING PHASE. In the context of two devices A and B along with the intermediate server C—there could be three possible options for alerting A:

1. C is aware of the proximity information between two users A and B after B is being reported positive and confirmation about that fact comes from a trusted and authorized source (e.g., health authority). Therefore, C arranges to send an alert to A.
2. C receives some data owned by B from other trusted and authorized source after B is being reported positive. C becomes aware of the proximity information between A and B only when A sends a query to check post which C arranges to send an alert to A.
3. C is aware of the list of individuals who have been tested positive and/or some identifiers from which their beacon packets can be identified. It periodically sends the information to all the devices. A matches the received information to find out if it came in close contact with any such individual and alerts its owner with the associated risk level (or risk score). There can also be another variation of the third approach where C is used as a post-box by both the parties (A and B) to secretly exchange the information about their proximity without revealing the identity of one party (say A) to the other parties (B and C). The post-box may have centralized or distributed implementation and the secrecy can be maintained via different cryptologic approaches and algorithms.

Among the three possible options mentioned above, the first option can be viewed as a centralized version, the third option as the decentralized version, and the second option as a hybrid of centralized and decentralized versions. Clearly, there are trade-offs for each of the versions and these trade-offs would be discussed in this book when we explain a concrete specification (like DP-3T) that may fall in any of these three architecture options.

IDENTIFIER. It must be noted that at the time of sharing of BLE packets between A and B, the payloads are expected not to reveal the identity of A or B in any way, i.e., from these packets, it would not be possible for either A's app or B's app (or any other party with malicious intent) to identify the device that has shared the packet. This aspect is usually achieved by using pseudorandom numbers as pseudonyms for the device which may either be a fixed identifier (not preferred as it would become easy to identify and track the device later) or a rotating identifier that changes in value every 15 min or so. There could also be ancillary data like exact or approximate time of the day, distance between the devices, relative speed, etc., stored along with the pseudonymous constantly rotating identifiers. Many times the expectations of privacy may need to be balanced against social responsibility or ethical considerations (individual's freedom vs collective good)—for example, if B is given freedom to decide about disclosure of his contact information for the past 14 days (from privacy perspective), there could be many other individuals adversely affected to not have the information about their possible infected states (which in turn would affect the collective well-being) in case B chooses not to disclose.

We would also discuss the adversarial scenarios and how in each of the situations, the possible attacks can be handled. It would also be important to consider certain fault scenarios and their implications on the system goals, e.g., if the BLE packets are somehow missed by any device, the completeness or comprehensiveness goal may get adversely impacted. The integration of the system architecture with the health authority is critical as in most of the proposals, there is an authorization step for B to upload his datasets with the confirmation indicator that he has been tested positive.

Finally, in technical architecture, it is important to point out that the digital contact tracing systems can be built in various layers. These layers are as follows:

- A specification that limits its scope at the communication protocol and data modeling level,
- A set of API libraries that are built on top of a communication protocol and data modeling layer,
- An app which uses proprietary or public-domain or open-source APIs,
- A framework or a system of apps, an interoperability infrastructure and a federated server systems to communicate across agencies and borders.

In each of these types of implementations, the designers may choose to make it open source or provide only a sample implementation without disclosing the backend source code.

1.5 Basics of Cryptology

For maintaining secrecy and privacy, we need cryptologic tools and our main motivation in this book is to have a look from that direction. We discuss a few primitives briefly in this section. For a more detailed introductory technical understanding, one may refer to [47].

1.5.1   Encryption

Encryption is the process of encoding information (plaintext) into a different form (ciphertext), through various means. Cryptographic encryption is implemented by using a function on the plaintext, along with another value, called a key. This encrypted data can then be decrypted using a decryption function on the cipher-text, possibly with the same or a different key. A secure encryption scheme is used to achieve privacy and confidentiality. In other words, an unauthorized user should not be able to get any information about the message from the encrypted message. Moreover, the secret key should be protected by any means, otherwise, the whole system will be completely broken. Cryptographic encryption can be broadly categorized into (i) public key (asymmetric) (ii) private key (symmetric) encryption, and (iii) hybrid encryption.

Public Key Encryption   Public key cryptography involves the use of two kinds of keys—a secret key which is not revealed to any entity other than the user to whom it belongs, and a public key which is known to everyone. Any user (sender) who requires to encrypt any information must use the public key of the receiver. The receiver can decrypt the ciphertext using his corresponding secret key to get back the original information. This is possible by mathematically linking the public and secret keys in a certain manner. Examples of public key encryption include the RSA algorithm [43], the ElGamal encryption [26], various elliptic curve-based encryptions [11, 30, 52], etc.

Symmetric Key Encryption   Unlike public key, it is assumed in symmetric key encryption processes that the two entities involved in the sharing of information (encryption and decryption) share the same secret key, which is unknown to any other entity. The common secret key is used for encryption as well as decryption algorithms. So, communication in symmetric key encryption is restricted to the authorized users, whereas in public key encryption, information can be sent to anybody having a public key and a secret key. However, symmetric key encryptions are much more efficient and lightweight. AES (a standardized algorithm by standard body of the USA, National Institute of Standards and Technology) is an example of symmetric key encryption which can encrypt 128-bit messages. CBC Encryption or counter mode encryptions are encryption algorithms which can encrypt messages of arbitrary length.

Hybrid Encryption   A hybrid scheme first determines a common shared secret key using a key-exchange mechanism (a close variant of a public key encryption). For example, the sender can encrypt session key and send it to the receiver. Using the session key, the users can then communicate through a more efficient symmetric key encryption algorithm. The Diffie-Hellman key-exchange protocol [23] is a popular example which is used in SSH [61] and TLS [21, 22, 42] protocols.

1.5.2 Hash and MAC

Hash Function   A cryptographic hash function takes as input, a message of arbitrary
   length, and returns a fixed-length output. Hash functions are usually very fast
   algorithms. So, they are also used as a preprocessor of some mechanisms that
   require the short fingerprint of a message that they produce.
   A cryptographic hash function has some desirable properties, which make it useful
   in various cryptographic constructions. These properties include collision resistance (it should be difficult to find two different messages with the same hash
   values), pre-image resistance or onewayness (it should be difficult to find a message which has a given hash value), etc. SHA2 and SHA3 are commonly used
   families of hash functions (where SHA stands for Secure Hashing Algorithms [9,
   29]). SHA3 is an NIST standard hash algorithm ([9]).
   Even though hash functions are public and usually do not take any secret input, one
   can always keep a part of the input as a secret key. Such hash functions are called
   keyed hash functions. Keyed hash functions achieve additional security such as
   unpredictability and pseudorandomness. Keyed hash functions are sometimes also
   called Message Authentication Codes (MACs).
Message Authentication Code   Message Authentication Codes (MACs) are cryptographic constructions used for authenticating messages. These codes take a
   message and a secret key as their input and give a tag as output (sometimes
   along with a ciphertext for the message, in which case it is called an authenticated
   encryption or AE). Like symmetric key encryption, the secret key is shared by two
   or more authorized users. In addition to authenticating the message (this property
   of a MAC is also called integrity), a MAC also ensures authenticity of the source.
   A rightly verified tag also ensures that the message has been sent by one of the
   authorized users (those users who share the common secret key). MAC constructions may (optionally) use various cryptographic objects such as hash functions,
   block ciphers (fixed size symmetric encryption), etc. Commonly known as MACs
   include the Wegman-Carter (WC) MAC [53], CBCMAC [8] and PMAC [10].

1.5.3 Digital Signature

A digital signature is a public key analog of MAC. Messages sent over certain channels may face a risk of being distorted due to reasons like a bad network or a malicious
entity. A digital signature is a value computed for each message input using a signing
key (which is secret and specific to users). This value is then used to authenticate the
sender and check the correctness (or integrity) of the message. Unlike in the case of
MACs, verification can be done by anyone who has the verification key corresponding to the signing key. As the public key in symmetric encryption, the verification
key is kept public.

Some digital signatures may also store other information about the message such as the origin, time of sending, etc. Digital signatures can also be applied for non-repudiation, by which, a sender who digitally signs a message cannot deny having signed it later.

Digital signatures are usually pre-processed by a secure hash function and implemented using the RSA [43] or other public key cryptosystems. It is easier to implement digital signatures for maintaining the authenticity and integrity of messages since these are very short values as compared to the far longer corresponding messages.

1.5.4 TRNG/PRBG/PRF

TRNG or True Random Number Generator   Most cryptographic constructions require the generation of random numbers or pseudorandom numbers for purposes of key generation, nonce generation, salt generation, etc. A true random number generator (TRNG) or randomness extractor works by taking some random sources as inputs and generates truly random outputs of some target size. A random source can be the current time or some other values which keeps on changing. A good cryptographic TRNG must be efficiently computable and statistically close to a truly random distribution.

PRBG or Pseudorandom Number Bit Generator   A cryptographic pseudorandom bit generator (PRBG) is a deterministic algorithm, quite similar to a TRNG. However, the input of PRBG is assumed to be true random and short. Moreover, it outputs a (comparatively far longer) string of pseudorandom bits. This output of a PRBG is called a pseudorandom bit sequence. A combination of TRNG and PRBG can produce arbitrary length pseudorandom or random-looking bit string. RC4 [44], SNOW4G [35] (used in 4G mobile encryption), ZUC [33] (Chinese standard) are some examples of PRBGs.

PRF or Pseudorandom Function   Usually, pseudorandom bit strings are generated in a sequential manner. Even though these algorithms are fast, we cannot randomly jump to the bits that are located far away. Pseudorandom function (PRF) are some examples of PRBG which can jump to a random position almost at no cost. Moreover, the bit strings can be generated in parallel which makes this primitive very useful in practice. In addition to the secret key, it also takes a position number as an input. It outputs a short random-looking bit sequence corresponding to the position. It is desirable that there is no correlation among the outputs computed for different positions. Pseudorandom function is also used to design key derivation function. Keyed hash functions and CMAC (NIST recommended pseudorandom function) are some examples of PRFs.

1.6   Contact Tracing Protocols

In this section, we present brief descriptions of some of the recent proposals and implemented solutions of digital contact tracing systems. We detail out these proposals and solutions in later chapters along with the analysis from a cryptographic point of view.

1.6.1   Entities and Modules

We now list down certain entities that are used in digital contact tracing systems. For a given system, not all entities may be applicable. Also, there could be certain overlap of features among the entities in a system and functionalities of multiple entities could be integrated into a single entity as well.

1. **User.** Any individual willing to participate in an automated contact tracing process having a device enabled with the interface required by the automated system (e.g., BLE, Bluetooth, WiFi, GPS, etc.) and its associated protocol stacks for communication can become a *user* of the system. To use the system, a user must install the app (or application), register, and start using the app in the recommended way as governed by digital contact tracing system.
2. **User-App.** This is the app that acts as the user interface to the digital contact tracing system. Depending on the design of the DCTS, it may perform different functionalities—including, but not limited to, the user registration, generation/downloading of proximity identifiers or downloading of keys from which such identifiers can be generated, sending and receiving packets to/from nearby devices running the same app, uploading of identifiers to some central or distributed server(s) and identification and intimation of the user's risk level (or risk-score) of getting infected with the help of other server(s). The terms like user and user-app (or app) may be used interchangeably.
3. **Central Server.** As described in Sect. 1.4.3, the central server (C) acts as the intermediate server between the devices A and B running the DCTS app and coming in proximity to each other. At the minimum, it is responsible for handling the registration, authentication, and deregistration of users. This is expected to be the case for a fully decentralized system. In a fully centralized DCTS, it may perform the functionalities of generating the pseudonymous identifiers to be used by the devices, hold the list of identifiers (sent/received) corresponding to the users who have been diagnosed positive and identify the risk levels (or risk-scores) of every user by referring to their (sent/received) proximity identifiers and matching those with the (sent/received) identifiers uploaded by the infected users' apps. At the implementation level, it may consist of multiple cloud-based servers and the administrative jurisdiction of these servers can be dependent upon their physical locations, associated authorities, and the laws of the land. There may also be a group of federated central servers that would manage the automated

contact tracing process in different countries or states or geographical regions while inter-operating among themselves to ensure a seamless movement of users across different regions.

4. **Distributed Servers.** Decentralized systems can use one or more distributed servers as intermediate server(s) between the two devices (**A** and **B**). The implementation of such Distributed Servers may be accomplished in the form of a public Bulletin Board Server, Distributed Hash Tables, Blockchain-Based Servers, etc. There should be a mechanism by which distributed servers and the central server (responsible for the user registration) communicate with each other to ensure the authentication of users at the time of accessing the Distributed Servers. The presence of Distributed Servers ensures privacy and security of sensitive proximity data and information shared by the users who have been diagnosed positive, in a way that no party (including the central administrative authority) may derive any useful information other than a user who needs to know his/her risk level (or risk-score) of being infected.

5. **Central Administrative Authority.** The main task of the Central Administrative Authority in a contact tracing system is the administration and management of the entire process, including the delegation of any administrative task to other authorities under its supervision. It is expected to have legal and administrative jurisdiction of central server and any other server used in the system. It may also fulfill other purposes such as estimating the spread of the disease, deciding upon the plan of actions in various scenarios of the spread, etc., or delegate such types of tasks to separate Epidemiological Authority.

6. **Health Authority.** A trusted Health Authority (HA), with its associated server and database, is required by the Central Administrative Authority as well as the apps to determine which users are infected. The HA should therefore ideally involve medical personnel and other health department officials. The responsibility of testing individuals would be the duty of such an authority. Depending upon the design of the system, either HA or the infected user (based on HA's validation) may upload the sent/received proximity identifiers to the Central/Distributed Server(s). The system should have checks and balances to prevent anyone from bypassing (or forging) the validation step that is mandatorily required to be done with the help of HA.

From the perspective of functionalities or phases, a digital contact tracing system may be divided into the following modules.

1. **Initial setup.** The roll-out of any automated contact tracing system starts with the initial setup phase. In this phase, the non-user entities like the central administrative authority, the health authority, the central server (including a system of federated central servers), the distributed servers (if present), etc., should establish the required symmetric and/or asymmetric keys for the purposes of exchanging information among themselves in an authenticated, private, and secured manner. A part of setup may also take place at the time of app installation by the users. Algorithms like hash functions, PRFs, PRGs, etc., that are used in various phases of the contact tracing process are also initialized in the setup phase.

2. **Registration and initialization.** An individual interested in joining the system as a user must first install the app (or application) on his/her device and create a valid login-id with the registration phase with which he/she would access the app in future. Once the installation and registration steps are completed, the app would initialize itself by contacting the backend server(s). These might include setting up certain authentication keys and/or encryption/decryption keys, downloading proximity identifiers from the backend server(s) or keys to generate such identifiers, setting up a local database at the device end, gathering some minimal information from the user (like the first part of his/her postal code), user's preferences (e.g., the look and feel theme of the app), etc., before the app can be effectively used for the purpose of automated contact tracing.

3. **Contact-Broadcast.** Once the registration and initialization phase is done, the user-app starts sending (in most of the cases broadcasting) proximity identifiers over a certain range so that the nearby devices running the app may receive these packets. This range is limited by the strength of the medium of broadcast (which makes BLE signals a very good option for such a medium). Every user-app is also designed to receive such proximity identifiers on a continuous basis if shared by other devices that are nearby. The physical interface through which such communication happens (like Bluetooth signal or Bluetooth scanning mode) must be kept *ON* for the app to run successfully.

4. **Reporting Infected Status to Server(s).** On being tested positive by the Health Authority (HA), a user would receive authentication to upload the relevant information to the server(s). Depending upon the legislative requirement of the concerned country or state, the user may be mandated or have an independent choice to upload the proximity identifiers sent/received in previous CTDays, where the parameter CTDays indicate the number of days for which the user is considered infectious (as per the guideline of the corresponding Health Authority).

5. **Risk-level (or risk-score) computation.** A user may receive exposure details from a server (Central or Distributed) or the user-app may download a list (or a subset) of proximity identifiers of infected users on the device and determine the exposure by matching the downloaded identifiers with those stored locally on the device. The form of identifiers downloaded from the server need not be the same as those stored on the device. Once the exposure details are known, the user-app may compute the risk level (or risk-score) of the user as per some risk-computation algorithm using other associated meta-data (like duration of exposures, distance between the devices as estimated from the signal strengths, etc.). The final result may be displayed to the user as the risk level (low, medium, high, etc.) or a risk-score (e.g., the probability of being infected). In some systems, the entire computation may take place at the backend and the user-app receives the final result and displays the same to the user. For the user, the next step could be getting tested or consulting a health professional or self-isolating for a certain number of days or do nothing depending upon the guideline from the local Health Authority. From the DCTS perspective also, there could be various options like preventing any further access of the user to the system unless he/she uploads a

validated test result or allowing a restricted access to the system or no change of access (again depending upon the action the user is advised to take based on his/her risk level/risk-score).

1.6.2   Centralized Versus Decentralized

In this section, we investigate the definitions of the two categories, referred to as centralized and decentralized systems (or protocols).

A natural definition of centralized could be those protocols in which the central server is present. The central server (C) can directly communicate to all the users (or user-apps), whereas two apps (A and B) can communicate with each other only when they are in close contact. All implemented and proposed solutions use a central server and hence by this definition, all existing systems can be categorized as centralized. **Is it possible to design a system that does not have an intermediate entity like the central server?**

This can be an interesting research question. In fact, Vaudenay has hinted at the possibility of using blockchain-based central database in his analysis [51] of DP-3T (Decentralized Privacy-Preserving Proximity Tracing) [24], a decentralized digital contact tracing protocol. Whenever there is a third entity, there would be a question of trust, security and privacy considerations for the new entity (in addition to the need of trust, security, and privacy for the existing entities coming in close proximity to each other). We would discuss in later chapters that there exists an inherent conflict among many of these considerations.

Here, we consider two different approaches that are used to define the centralized and decentralized protocols. In one approach, we look at the role that the central server plays in the contact broadcast phase of the protocol, while in the other, the categorization is based upon the core challenges that the protocol aims to solve.

1.6.2.1   Centralized or Decentralized: Nature of Communications of a Protocol

Currently, the cryptographic community defines the centralized and decentralized categories based on how the proximity identifiers are derived or generated.

1. If the proximity identifiers are known to (or could be derived from a key supplied by) the central server then we call the protocol centralized. The prominent examples are BlueTrace, NTK, and ROBERT.
2. On the other hand, if the proximity identifiers are not known to the central server, then we call the protocol decentralized. This means, for decentralized protocols, the proximity identifiers are generated only by the user-app (or the client-side application run at the user's device end) and only in the event a user is tested positive, some of these identifiers may become known to the central server (how-

ever, in some protocols even that may not happen). So a decentralized protocol can run the contact broadcast phase without any help from the central server. The examples of decentralized protocols are DP-3T, Apple-Google, PACT (East and West), TCN, Pronto-C2, DESIRE, Epione, protocol proposed by the IST group, etc.

1.6.2.2 Centralized or Decentralized: Nature of Goal of a Protocol

We can also categorize the protocols by looking at the problems that the protocol aims to solve.

Here, we identify two types of goals or problems-

1. In one of the types, a centralized protocol is one in which the central server can trace all the contacts of a positively-diagnosed user as soon as he/she reports the status (of being infected) to the system. The protocols for which this would not be feasible would be categorized as decentralized. In this approach, BlueTrace, Aarogya Setu would be classified as centralized and almost all other systems would fall under the category of decentralized.
2. In another approach, we consider a protocol decentralized if the central server does not have any information about the "close contact" events. Therefore in such systems, the risk level (or risk-score) of a user can not be computed by the central server. However, the central server may have some information (e.g., the proximity identifiers sent in the last CT days) about the users who have been diagnosed positive. Hence, DP-3T, Apple-Google, PACT (East coast and West coast) can be categorized as decentralized protocols whereas BlueTrace, NTK, ROBERT, etc. would fall under the bucket of centralized protocols.

From these discussions, it would be apparent that there could be several other possible types of categorizations as well for defining the centralized and decentralized protocols. One may also create a hybrid of some of the above approaches and define that as a new categorization. For example, we may define a system as decentralized only when the central server does not play any role in generating the proximity identifiers, has no role to identify the "close contact" events, does not compute the risk level (or risk-score) of a user and has no direct knowledge of infected users. In this approach, DESIRE will be classified as a decentralized protocol but DP-3T, Apple-Google, etc., would be viewed as centralized protocols. It must be pointed out that a protocol that is considered decentralized as per its role (at the time of contact broadcast event) can potentially be converted to a decentralized one according to the type of problem it solves, however, a protocol where the proximity identifiers are generated by the central server cannot be converted so easily to the decentralized version.

1.6.3 Security and Privacy Assumptions

Certain reasonable assumptions must be made about the security and integrity of these entities against attacks from a malicious entity or other adversaries. This not only requires notions of trust but also permissions for communication to be built for these entities.

1. The health authority may only provide information about positive users to the server. The health authority is assumed to be a fully trusted entity, as otherwise, the absence of reliable testing and infection data would render the entire exercise pointless.
2. The central server may not necessarily be trusted, and it could prove useful to consider some attacks from a malicious server.
3. Any two user-apps may communicate with each other only if in close contact. Finally, although users cannot be trusted at all, user apps may or may not be trusted.
4. All communications from a user to the server and from the server to the health authority are carried out over a secure channel (e.g., by using TLS protocol). On the other hand, communication between users cannot be considered to take place over a secure channel, which renders it vulnerable to tapping, but it is not tamperable.

SEMI- HONEST AND ACTIVE MODEL OF ADVERSARY. These assumptions about the powers an adversary may possess over each of these entities leads to the following two distinctions: In a *semi-honest model*, an adversary will follow the protocol honestly, but gain information from this honest transcript, whereas in an *active model*, an adversary has the power to gain extra information through dishonest means. If the semi-honest model is a preference, the contact tracing app must be installed in a TPM (Trusted Platform Module); in case the enforcement of a TPM is not possible, the active model must be allowed. We may have a hybrid of the above two models where some simple computation can be assumed to be done honestly and the rest can be done arbitrarily by an adversary. This could be a reasonable assumption as the implementation of TPM can be costly and the cost could depend on the computation which would be done in TPM.

1.7 Some Examples of Contact Tracing Protocols

In this section, we provide brief descriptions of some digital contact tracing protocols/systems that have already been launched or have been proposed. The detailed descriptions and analyses of the protocols and systems are presented in Chaps. 2 and 3 under the categorization of centralized and decentralized systems respectively. The intent here is to provide the reader with a glimpse of the variety of approaches and not an exhaustive listing of the launched or proposed systems.

1.7.1   The TraceTogether System (BlueTrace Protocol)

TraceTogether is the first digital contact tracing system (DCTS) that was deployed at a country level for automated contact tracing of SARS-CoV-2 infection. It was developed by Singapore's Government Technology Agency and was launched on 20 March 2020 to supplement the centralized contact tracing effort of the Ministry of Health. The source code of the app was later released to the open-source community as OpenTrace along with the design specification of the protocol (called BlueTrace) on top of which the app had been developed. The detailed documentation (including a white paper) about the BlueTrace protocol is available in its official website [7, 13].

In this protocol, the proximity identifiers (called the temporary IDs) are generated by the backend server (or the central server). A central database, hosted in the cloud-based secured backend server and administered by the Ministry of Health, keeps track of the permanent ID of every device that is generated at the time of registration against a phone number. When a user of the app (say B) is found to be infected, a contact tracer will reach out and ask him to securely upload the temporary IDs received by his device (say B) in the last 14 days to the central server. In the backend, the received temporary IDs would be analyzed to identify the permanent IDs of the users corresponding to those temporary IDs. The Ministry of Health personnel would next contact the individuals who came in close contact with B, by referring to the phone numbers stored in the central database against their permanent IDs. The usual process that is followed in case of manual contact tracing would then be followed for these individuals.

Based on our discussion from the previous section on the classification of automated contact tracing systems, we can categorize the TraceTogether (as well as OpenTrace and BlueTrace) under the centralized category.

Australian Government has recently launched the COVIDSafe app that has been built on top of the BlueTrace protocol [19]. At the implementation level, there are certain differences between TraceTogether and COVIDSafe. In both the systems, the apps can run seamlessly in the background mode on Android phones. However, the apps can be used in Apple phones successfully only when running in the foreground mode which is not a convenient option for the users. In case of COVIDSafe, any uploading of proximity data to the central database can be done when the user who has been diagnosed positive gives consent to the health authority.

1.7.2   Aarogya Setu

The Government of India has launched Aarogya Setu [1, 2] as "...a digital service, primarily a mobile application, developed by the Government of India and is aimed at protecting the citizens during SARS-CoV-2. It is designed to augment the initiatives of the Government of India by informing the people of their potential risk of SARS-

CoV-2 infection and the best practices to be followed to stay healthy, as well as providing them relevant and curated medical advisories, as per MoHFW and ICMR guidelines, pertaining to the SARS-CoV-2 pandemic." It has been developed by the National Informatics Center (NIC)

As per the FAQ [2], the salient features of this system are:

- Automatic contact tracing using Bluetooth,
- Self-assessment test based on ICMR guidelines,
- Risk status of user,
- Updates, advisory, and best practices related to SARS-CoV-2,
- Geo location-based SARS-CoV-2 statistics,
- Nationwide SARS-CoV-2 statistics,
- Emergency SARS-CoV-2 helpline contacts,
- List of ICMR approved labs with SARS-CoV-2 testing facilities,
- e-Pass integration, and
- Support for 12 languages.

The risk status of a user is indicated by four different colors where "Green" signifies Low Risk, "Yellow" means Moderate Risk, "Orange" indicates High Risk, while "Red" implies SARS-CoV-2-positive status. The digital signature of every interaction is created by recording the time, the duration, the proximity, and the location. The contact data is stored for 14 days in the device and the risk computation is done at the app end by referring to the list of identifiers sent by the infected users in the last 14 days and cross-checking the local database at the device end for any possible matches.

The app is available for iOS, Android, KaiOS operating systems and it requires Bluetooth as well as GPS protocols to be enabled for its effective functioning. Identifiers get shared through Bluetooth messages between two devices that come in close proximity to each other. The system tries to check whether the user has come in close contact with SARS-CoV-2-infected person by cross-referencing the proximity data against a centralized database of known cases.

1.7.3   ROBERT and DESIRE

Researchers from two institutions, namely France's Inria and Germany's Fraunhofer, have come up with a digital contact tracing protocol which they have named as ROBust and privacy-presERving proximity tracing protocol (ROBERT). These two institutes are also members of Pan-European Privacy-Preserving Proximity Tracing (PEPP-PT) project.

A detailed set of documents including a high-level summary illustrated example and a detailed specification have been shared by the team in Github repository [45]. In a way, ROBERT lies between the centralized and decentralized systems as there are some aspects in which it is similar to a centralized protocol (like BlueTrace), while in some other features, it behaves more like a decentralized protocol. The proximity identifiers (called EphIDs) in ROBERT are generated by the central server and shared with the devices that eventually use the same in the contact broadcast phase.

When a user is tested positive, with his/her permission and with the authorization of the Health Authority, the entire list of EphIDs that it received from other devices that came in close proximity in the last 14 days—gets uploaded to the central server (in this way, it is similar to BlueTrace protocol). The detection of possible exposure events and the computation of risk scores are done in the central server.

We position this protocol in between centralized and decentralized categories because the main function of identifying potential exposure events is divided into two parts. On one hand, the detection of proximity of an infected user (B) with another (who is not yet known to be infected) user (A) is done at the central server end, while on the other, the discovery of the possible exposure is done by A (the mobile device of A) when it explicitly requests the server for such information.

DESIRE protocol has been proposed as an evolution of the ROBERT protocol by the PRIVATICS project team from Inria, France. It is a more decentralized protocol than ROBERT. In DESIRE, the mobile devices generate the EphIDs independently without the help of the server and store those in such a fashion (using a non-interactive key exchange protocol) that the IDs can be transparently matched at the server end to identify the possible close-contact events without any possibility of recovering the original pseudorandom IDs that got exchanged between the devices when they came in close proximity to each other.

1.7.4 East Coast PACT

This is the acronym for Private Automated Contact Tracing (PACT) protocol that has been proposed by the joint group of academicians/researchers/professionals in the US from MIT, ACLU, Boston University, American Civil Liberties Union, Brown University, MIT Lincoln Laboratory, Weizmann Institute, and Thinking Cyber-security.

The detailed specification is available at [38] and is licensed under the Creative Commons Attribution 4.0 License.

This is also a decentralized protocol with a lot of overlap in basic features with DP-3T. In fact, the specification has highlighted that there exist a number of similarities with some other proposals as well—including, the West Coast PACT [39], the strawman protocol from Covid-Watch project [32, 46] and the Canetti et al. protocol [15].

One may also refer to some other references in this regard at [16, 28, 40, 48].

1.7.5 Apple-Google Exposure Notification Framework

Apple and Google have jointly worked and developed a protocol specification and an API framework [4] for an exposure notification system that can be accessed by an authorized app in Android and iOS platforms. The specification is hugely influenced by the DP-3T protocol and the TCN protocol by Covid Watch [20]. The primary differentiator of this protocol and API framework is that it can be used by apps running in the background mode in both Android and iOS devices which is not the case for any other launched systems so far. At this point of time, a number of countries (including the UK) have developed automated contact tracing systems using the Apple-Google framework.

1.8 Conclusion

In this chapter, we introduce the basic understanding of contact tracing protocols. Not only the technical points we also try to touch upon the social issues given the unexpected SARS-CoV-2 pandemic. It is quite evident that all the problems can never be solved by digital and automated contact tracing protocols using smartphones. However, technology can always help in fighting a virus, at least in its limited capacity. The success of technology is always connected to social and political will. Thus, while not sufficient, technology is necessary to fight this virus and that is why so many protocols are arriving in a short time. We must accept that in this effort we could not touch upon all the proposals, but the important ones are listed in this chapter. We also provide a brief overview of related cryptologic primitives. With this background, we continue with more detailed technical aspects in the following chapters. In the next chapter, we concentrate mostly on the proposals that are centralized in nature.

References

1. Aarogya Setu App. https://www.mygov.in/aarogya-setu-app/.
2. Aarogya Setu FAQs. Accessed 26 May 2020. https://static.mygov.in/rest/s3fs-public/mygov_159056978751307401.pdf.
3. Altuwaiyan, T., Hadian, M., & Liang, X. (2018). EPIC: Efficient privacy-preserving contact tracing for infection detection. In *2018 IEEE International Conference on Communications (ICC)*, Kansas City, MO, 2018 (pp. 1–6). https://ieeexplore.ieee.org/document/8422886.
4. Apple and Google. Privacy-preserving contact tracing. https://www.apple.com/covid19/contacttracing.
5. Apuzzo, M., Gebrekidan, S., & Kirkpatrick, D. D. (2020). How the world missed Covid-19's silent spread? Retrieved June 28, 2020. https://timesofindia.indiatimes.com/world/europe/how-the-world-missed-covid-19s-silent-spread/articleshow/76673535.cms.
6. Ariel Bogle. COVIDSafe's effectiveness on iPhone in question as Government releases coronavirus contact tracing app. Retrieved April 26, 2020, https://www.abc.net.au/news/2020-04-26/coronavirus-tracing-app-covidsafe-apple-iphone-covid-19/12187448.
7. Bay, J., Kek, J., Tan, A., Hau, C. S., Yongquan, L., Tan, J., & Quy, T. A. BlueTrace: A privacy-preserving protocol for community-driven contact tracing across borders. https://bluetrace.io/static/bluetrace_whitepaper-938063656596c104632def383eb33b3c.pdf.
8. Bellare, M., Kilian, J., & Rogaway, P. (2000). The security of the cipher block chaining message authentication code. *Journal of Computer and System Sciences, 61*(3), 362–399.

9. Bertoni, G., Daemen, J., Peeters, M., & Van Assche, G. (2013). Keccak. In T. Johansson & P. Q. Nguyen (Eds.), *Advances in Cryptology - EUROCRYPT 2013* (pp. 313–314). Berlin: Springer.
10. Black, J., & Rogaway, P. (2000). Cbc macs for arbitrary-length messages: The three-key constructions. In *Proceedings of the 20th Annual International Cryptology Conference on Advances in Cryptology*, CRYPTO '00 (pp. 197–215). Berlin: Springer.
11. Blake, I., Seroussi, G., & Smart, N. (1999). *Elliptic Curves in Cryptography. London Mathematical Society Lecture Note Series.* Cambridge: Cambridge University Press.
12. BLE: Overview of COVID-19 contact tracing using BLE. https://blog.google/documents/57/Overview_of_COVID-19_Contact_Tracing_Using_BLE.pdf.
13. BlueTrace Protocol: Privacy-preserving cross-border contact tracing. https://bluetrace.io/.
14. Bluetooth Low Energy. Smart or Version 4.0+ of the Bluetooth specification. bluetooth.com. Archived from the original on 10 March 2017 (Accessed via https://web.archive.org/web/20170310111443/, https://www.bluetooth.com/what-is-bluetooth-technology/how-it-works/low-energy).
15. Canetti, R., Trachtenberg, A., & Varia, M. Anonymous collocation discovery: Harnessing privacy to tame the coronavirus. arXiv:2003.13670.
16. Cho, H., Ippolito, D., & Yu, Y. W. Contact tracing mobile Apps for COVID-19 privacy considerations and related trade-offs. arXiv:2003.11511.
17. Contact Tracing – Wikipedia. https://en.wikipedia.org/wiki/Contact_tracing.
18. Contact Tracing for COVID-19. https://www.cdc.gov/coronavirus/2019-ncov/php/contact-tracing/contact-tracing-plan/contact-tracing.html.
19. COVIDSafe app. https://www.health.gov.au/resources/apps-and-tools/covidsafe-app.
20. Covid Watch. https://covid-watch.org/.
21. Dierks, T., & Allen, C. (1999). RFC2246: The TLS Protocol Version 1.0.
22. Dierks, T., & Rescorla, E. (2006). The Transport Layer Security (TLS) protocol version 1.1. RFC 4346. Archived from the original on 2017-12-24.
23. Diffie, W., & Hellman, M. (1976). New Directions in Cryptography. *IEEE Transactions on Information Theory, 22*(6), 644–654.
24. DP-3T White Paper. https://github.com/DP-3T/documents, https://github.com/DP-3T/documents/blob/master/DP3T%20White%20Paper.pdf.
25. Ebola Report: Tracing Contacts. https://www.cdc.gov/about/ebola/tracing-contacts.html.
26. El Gamal, T. (1985). A public key cryptosystem and a signature scheme based on discrete logarithms. In *Proceedings of CRYPTO 84 on Advances in Cryptology* (pp. 10–18). Berlin: Springer.
27. Farrahi, K., Emonet, R., & Cebrian, M. (2014). Epidemic contact tracing via communication traces. PLOS ONE. Retrieved May 1, 2014, https://journals.plos.org/plosone/article?id=10.1371/journal.pone.0095133.
28. Gvili, Y. Security analysis of the COVID-19 contact tracing specifications by Apple Inc. and Google Inc. https://eprint.iacr.org/2020/428.pdf.
29. Handschuh, H. (2011). Sha-0, sha-1, sha-2 (secure hash algorithm). In H. C. A. van Tilborg, & S. Jajodia (Eds.), *Encyclopedia of Cryptography and Security*, (2nd Ed., pp. 1190–1193). Springer.
30. Hankerson, D., & Menezes, A. (2011). *Elliptic curve cryptography* (p. 397). Boston: Springer US.
31. Hart, M. B., & Yarwood, T. (2020) Explainer: What is contact tracing and how does it help limit the coronavirus spread? Retrieved March 27, 2020, https://theconversation.com/explainer-what-is-contact-tracing-and-how-does-it-help-limit-the-coronavirus-spread-134228.
32. Ingle, M., White, T., Becker-Mayer, I., Petrie, J., Szabo, Z., Blank, D., Colligan, J., Hittle, M., Fenwick, R., Nash, O., Nguyen, V., Schwaber, J., Veeraghanta, A., Voloshin, M., Von Arx, S., & Xue, H. (2020) Slowing the spread of infectious diseases using crowdsourced data. Retrieved March 20, 2020, https://www.covid-watch.org/, https://www.covid-watch.org/article#contactTracing.
33. Jing, J., Liu, Z., Zhang, L., & Pan, W. (2010). Efficient pipelined stream cipher ZUC algorithm in FPGAC.

34. Khalid, A., & Shendruk, A. (2020). How bluetooth could unleash the world's largest experiment in digital contact tracing. Retrieved April 16, 2020, https://qz.com/1838625/how-bluetooth-could-power-a-global-experiment-in-contact-tracing/.
35. Madani, M., Benkhaddra, I., Tanougast, C., Chitroub, S., & Siéler, L. (2017). Digital implementation of an improved LTE stream cipher snow-3G based on hyperchaotic PRNG. *Security and Communication Networks, 2017*, 5746976:1–5746976:15.
36. McDonnell, T. (2020). Is it too soon for a "CoronaPass" immunity app? Retrieved April 16, 2020 https://qz.com/1838764/is-it-too-soon-for-immunity-passports/.
37. Muller, J. (2019). *Smartphone penetration as share of population in Singapore 2017–2023.* Statista. Retrieved Sep 9, 2019, https://www.statista.com/statistics/625441/smartphone-user-penetration-in-singapore/.
38. PACT protocol specification - version 0.1 (4/8/2020). https://pact.mit.edu/wp-content/uploads/2020/04/The-PACT-protocol-specification-ver-0.1.pdf.
39. PACT: Privacy-sensitive protocols and mechanisms for mobile contact tracing. https://arxiv.org/abs/2004.03544.
40. Privacy-preserving contact tracing - Apple and Google. https://www.apple.com/covid19/contacttracing.
41. PTI London. Nearly 200 genetic mutations identified in SARS-CoV2. Retrieved May 06, 2020, https://www.thehindubusinessline.com/news/science/nearly-200-genetic-mutations-identified-in-sars-cov2/article31520645.ece.
42. Rescorla, E. (2018). The Transport Layer Security (TLS) Protocol Version 1.3. RFC 8446.
43. Rivest, R. L., Shamir, A., & Adleman, L. (1978). A method for obtaining digital signatures and public-key cryptosystems. *Communications of the ACM, 21*(2), 120–126.
44. Rivest, R. L., & Schuldt, J. C. N. (2016). Spritz—a spongy rc4-like stream cipher and hash function. Cryptology ePrint Archive, Report 2016/856. https://eprint.iacr.org/2016/856.
45. ROBERT: ROBust and privacy-presERving proximity Tracing - Inria, France and Fraunhofer AISEC, Germany. https://github.com/ROBERT-proximity-tracing/documents.
46. Specification and reference implementation of the TCN Protocol for decentralized, privacy-preserving contact tracing. https://github.com/TCNCoalition/TCN.
47. Stinson, D. R. (2002). *Cryptography - Theory and practice* (2nd ed.). Boca Raton: Chapman & Hall/CRC.
48. Tang, Q. Privacy-preserving contact tracing: Current solutions and open questions. arXiv:2004.06818.
49. Townsend, K. Introduction to bluetooth low energy. Adafruit Learning System. https://cdn-learn.adafruit.com/downloads/pdf/introduction-to-bluetooth-low-energy.pdf.
50. Townsend, K., Cufi, C., Akiba, & Davidson, R. (2014). *Getting started with bluetooth low energy.* Sebastopol: Oreilly. https://www.oreilly.com/library/view/getting-started-with/9781491900550/ch01.html.
51. Vaudenay, S. Analysis of DP-3T between Scylla and Charybdis. https://eprint.iacr.org/2020/399.pdf.
52. Washington, L. C. (2008). *Elliptic Curves: Number Theory and Cryptography, Second Edition* (2nd ed.). London: Chapman and Hall (CRC).
53. Wegman, M. N., & Carter, L. (1981). New hash functions and their use in authentication and set equality. *Journal of Computer and System Sciences, 22*, 265–279.
54. Wiki: Compartmental models in epidemiology. https://en.wikipedia.org/wiki/Compartmental_models_in_epidemiology.
55. Wolfel, R. et al. (2020). Virological assessment of hospitalized patients with COVID-2019. *Nature, 581*, 465–469. https://www.nature.com/articles/s41586-020-2196-x.
56. World Health Organization. https://www.who.int/.
57. World Health Organization. https://www.who.int/news-room/q-a-detail/contact-tracing.
58. World Health Organization. https://www.who.int/docs/default-source/coronaviruse/situation-reports/20200402-sitrep-73-covid-19.pdf?sfvrsn=5ae25bc7_2.
59. World Health Organization. How long does the virus survive on surfaces? https://www.who.int/news-room/q-a-detail/q-a-coronaviruses.

60. World Health Organization. Transmission of COVID-19 by asymptomatic cases. Retrieved June 11, 2020, http://www.emro.who.int/health-topics/corona-virus/transmission-of-covid-19-by-asymptomatic-cases.html.
61. Ylonen, T. (1996). SSH - Secure Login Connections over the Internet (pp. 37–42).
62. Zhang, R., Zhang, J., Zhang, Y., Sun, J., & Yan, G. (2013). Privacy-preserving profile matching for proximity-based mobile social networking. *IEEE Journal on Selected Areas in Communications*, *31*(9), 656–668. https://ieeexplore.ieee.org/document/6544548.

Chapter 2
Centralized Systems

Abstract Digital Contact Tracing (DCT) protocols and systems usually rely on close-range communications between handheld devices (like smartphones and tablets), primarily through a Bluetooth Low Energy (BLE) interface and a client-server mode of communication between the apps installed on the devices and the backend server(s). Depending upon the role played by the backend server(s), DCT protocols and systems are usually classified as centralized or decentralized. In Chap. 1, we have discussed some of the competing ways of classifying systems, eventually settling with the following broad-level understanding: for the scope of this book, we shall consider a system (or a protocol) centralized if the backend server(s) plays (or play) a dominant role in deciding the risk level (or risk-score) of an individual being infected. This chapter focuses on centralized systems and protocols like BlueTrace, TraceTogether, COVIDSafe, ROBERT etc. It also presents a generalized framework of centralized systems before going deep into the specific systems. The chapter ends with discussions on systems that lie in between the centralized and decentralized categories, thus setting the stage for decentralized systems in Chap. 3.

2.1 Introduction

The central server of any digital contact tracing system may have access to certain personal or personally identifiable information (like phone number, postal code etc.) of the user. If these datasets are not stored in an encrypted form, there is a significant risk of loss of users' privacy. Hence, all DCT systems and protocols proposed so far make use of pseudonymous identifiers. These identifiers can be of two types—one associated permanently with an instance of user-app right from the registration phase, and the other generated for the purpose of sharing proximity identifiers between two nearby user-apps/devices. If the latter type of identifiers does not change over time, a malicious entity may be able to track the movement of a particular user by capturing

P. Chakraborty et al., *Contact Tracing in Post-Covid World*,
Indian Statistical Institute Series,
https://doi.org/10.1007/978-981-15-9727-5_2

the unchanging proximity identifier emitted by the user-app and then associating it with the user's device through some other means (e.g. through photographic or video recording of the user in some location). In order to avoid tracking through similar methods, all DCT systems and protocols are designed to change their proximity identifiers frequently.

In most centralized systems, the central server is usually responsible for generating these identifiers. This (possibly accompanied by other capabilities it may possess) may provide the central server in a centralized system to become aware of the list of contacts of an infected user; a compilation of such data from multiple users can be utilized to generate a social graph of users. Central servers and databases must be provided the highest level of data security so as to avoid any leakage or compromise of sensitive user-data.

2.1.1 Background

In Chap. 1, we have described the rationale behind the division of digital contact tracing systems in two categories—centralized and decentralized. We have also pointed out that due to the multiple ways of defining centralized or decentralized schemes, some centralized systems have many decentralized features and likewise, almost all decentralized systems, with certain functionalities delegated to the backend server, could be viewed as partially centralized systems. With more and more DCT systems being proposed, one may expect the eventual emergence of a continuum between the two extremes of fully centralized and fully decentralized systems, irrespective of how one may choose to define the categories.

This chapter starts with a description of the centralized protocol BlueTrace, followed by descriptions of COVIDSafe, PEPP-PT NTK and Aarogya Setu, and eventually concluding with a detailed study of a protocol that lies in the middle of the centralized-to-decentralized continuum, called ROBERT, and its evolved successor DESIRE, which moves further away from centralization and towards the decentralized end of this continuum. In the absence of standard design specifications or a documentation on the cryptographic algorithms used for centralized systems like PEPP-PT, NHS_COVID-19 app etc., we have provided high-level descriptions instead of detailed system analyses.

2.1.2 Characteristics of Centralized Systems

Let us now discuss the typical characteristics of a centralized digital contact tracing system. Centralized systems are designed as a natural extension of the manual contact tracing process, in which human contact tracers reach out to the primary, secondary or tertiary contacts after interviewing the index cases and provide the concerned individuals with guidance, health advice and counseling (wherever required). Centralized systems also act as the nerve center of the entire operation by managing, controlling and limiting the spread of the infectious disease. The common characteristics of almost all centralized systems are as follows.

- A centralized agency like the Health Department or the Ministry of Health assumes the authority on the entire digital contact tracing system (including the data stored in the server).
- The backend server(s) and central database(s) are viewed as trusted entities that can securely manage the user-specific data and maintain the privacy of the users.
- If a user tests positive, then he/she would be expected to upload one's proximity identifiers (shared by one's user-app with the neighbouring devices and/or received from such devices over the last 14 days or so) to the backend server(s).
- The backend server(s) help (either proactively or based on request) in the identification of contacts who could be at risk of infection.
- The contact data is used by the backend to either reach out to the person (if evaluated to be at risk of being infected) via a human contact tracer or update the corresponding risk level (or the risk-score) to the central database(s), which can be retrieved by the user-app from time to time.
- In case the security of the server data is compromised and sensitive data of users fall in the hands of malicious actors or groups, the extent of damage could be significant. This makes the minimization of collection of personal or personally identifiable data a critical evaluation parameter in centralized systems and protocols.
- Epidemiological analysis can be done easily from the data stored in the backend server.
- It becomes important to track how the backend data is stored by the service provider (like Google Cloud Services, Amazon Web Services etc.) in the data centers, so that no other entity (e.g. the government of another country) may have legal rights or control on the data.

Extensibility beyond one country, jurisdiction or region: Since the backend server acts as the nerve center of the entire system, it becomes easy to design a federated system of cooperating and trusting servers that may communicate with each other to manage the contact tracing process across regional or national boundaries.

Ease of modification: Since most critical operations including evaluation of the *at-risk* or *not at-risk* status of users are carried out centrally, it may become easier in centralized systems to roll out changes, bug-fixes and enhancements (e.g. modification of the risk-scoring algorithm) as compared to decentralized systems.

2.1.2.1 Common Cryptographic Primitives

We now take a look at some important cryptographic primitives in centralized systems.

- **Proximity identifiers.** Frequently changing pseudonymous and pseudorandom identifiers that are exchanged between the user-apps when any two devices come near each other.
- **Encryption and authentication keys.** These keys are required during device-to device, device-to-server or server-to-server communications. They may be symmetric or asymmetric, and can be exchanged by following any interactive or non-interactive key-exchange protocol.
- **Permanent identifiers.** A permanent identifier may be uniquely associated with each user-app and may correspond to other personal or personally identifiable information (like a user's phone number).
- **Other codes.** This may include an encrypted country code, encrypted epoch number (signifying a specific start and end time) etc.

2.2 A General Framework of Centralized Protocol

A general centralized protocol for contact tracing is mainly characterized by the interaction of various entities with the central server. User-apps receive proximity identifier(s) from the server (in some cases, users may locally generate these identifiers), which they broadcast or exchange with other user-apps when in proximity. An infected user's app uploads one's received (and/or sent) identifiers to the server after authorization from a health authority, and another user intending to check one's exposure status may either wait to receive a direct notification from the server (or from a person in case of a *human-in-the-loop* system like TraceTogether), or query the server by passing its sent (and/or received) identifiers and determine the risk level (or risk-score) of its user as computed by the server. The central server(s) of a centralized system thus plays a more prominent role in comparison to the central server(s) of decentralized protocols.

In Chap. 1, we have described different phases of a DCTS. Here, we focus on the features that are specific to centralized systems.

1. **Registration and Initialization Phase.** At the time of registration and initialization, the user-app may receive the first set of proximity identifiers to be used (or the keys from which such identifiers can be generated) from the server in a centralized DCT system. It may continue to receive new sets of proximity identifiers in a batch-mode after fixed time-intervals (e.g. after every 24 h).
2. **Contact-Broadcast Phase.** There is no difference between centralized and decentralized systems in this phase.
3. **Reporting Phase.** In a centralized system, the app of a positively diagnosed user uploads the received (and/or sent) proximity identifiers (for, say, the past 14 days) to the central server (upon user's consent and with the mandatory authorization by the health authority).
4. **Risk-level (or Risk-score) Computation Phase.** In some centralized systems, the server proactively identifies user(s) who may be at-risk of infection and notifies

them. This step may also be human-led as in the case of TraceTogether. Alternatively, the server computes the risk level (or risk-score) when a user-app sends an explicit request to compute the exposure risk.

Vaudenay proposes an interesting way of distinction between centralized and decentralized contact tracing systems in [39]. If the server generates and provides users with their ephemeral identifiers or if (possibly only infected) users communicate their own identifiers (or keys, pseudonyms, etc.) that allow the server to compute their identities, then the system is a centralized one. *ROBERT* [19, 20], *TraceTogether* [37], *Arogya Setu* [2–4], etc. are examples of centralized contact tracing systems.

2.2.1   A Naive Centralized Solution

A Hypothetical Insecure Protocol: If privacy were not a concern, it would be easy to build a smartphone-based centralized protocol. Whenever two phones come close enough (which can be detected through a simple Bluetooth program), both phones determine the other's identity (say phone number). This information is pushed to the server on a regular basis. Whenever an individual (say A) is reported positive for SARS-CoV-2, the server can determine which other users were close to A. This does not provide any user privacy to other users as well as to the server, as personal identities (such as phone numbers) are disclosed to everybody involved in the process. Moreover, it also reveals the social interaction graph (much bigger than interaction with a positive patient) to the server.

SECURITY REQUIREMENT: (**User privacy**) Any information related to the user's identity should not be disclosed to the other without the consent of the owner.

This protocol allows server and users to get information beyond what is needed for the purpose of contact tracing. The following protocol realizes only a slightly higher level of sophistication than the last, and can provide privacy amongst users, which the previous method failed to achieve.

1. Each device would continually broadcast some random numbers and store these numbers locally.
2. Any device (say B), which is close to a device (say A), receives A's random numbers and stores them.
3. On a regular basis, all devices will push their identity along with all the random numbers that they sent as well as received.
4. Whenever user A is reported positive, its identity details are sent to the server. The server can then easily identify all users (or devices), who were in closed contact of A.

Another simple alternative for the above protocol could be where the random numbers are generated (may be through a cryptographic primitive with a trapdoor) by the server. Every day, the central server push those numbers to users and the users broadcast those numbers through Bluetooth to all users who got close contact. Clearly, privacy between two users is achieved (as they only receive some random numbers). However, the server can easily track all individuals. In particular, the server still knows the social interaction of all users. That means, although there is privacy against users, there is no privacy against the server. This leads to a natural categorization of privacy of a user into two types:

1. privacy against users and
2. privacy against the central server or central administration.

However, one may allow the central server to identify all users who may have been in close contact with some SARS-CoV-2-positive user within a certain time window. Depending on situations, infrastructure, awareness of people of a country, one can consider some relaxed notion of privacy against the central administration. We call them centralized protocols. However, it is very important to know the entire extent of information that the server can gather even after behaving dishonestly. From cryptographic and privacy angles, it should not be relaxed to a level where surveillance of users is possible.

Restricting the data shared with the server: In the previous protocol, all the random numbers sent and received by each device are shared with the central server. This causes a significant loss of privacy as the central server can easily construct a social graph of the users at any point of time with the information shared by all the devices. On the other hand, if the server comes to know only the random numbers that are broadcast by all the devices (and not the ones that are received by the devices), it would not be able to deduce who came in contact with whom (and when) unless someone is tested positive, at which stage it would come to know of the random numbers received by the infected user's device so that it may help in identifying or notifying the at-risk individuals.

2.2.2 Attack Scenarios

Examination of possible attack scenarios is important for analyzing the security of the specific systems and protocols in this chapter. A more elaborate version of these scenarios is presented in Chap. 4. Here, we divide the attacks under three broad categories, namely (1) Integrity Attacks (2) Privacy Attacks and (3) Non-cryptographic Attacks.

2.2.2.1 Integrity Attacks

The integrity of a contact tracing system may be compromised through false positive alerts, i.e. when a user's device triggers an alert in spite of the user not having been in the proximity of a user (in, say, the past 14 days) who is later diagnosed as positive. Called a *trolling attack* by Yaron Gvili [18], a simple way to generate false positives is one in which an adversary "borrows" the device of a user diagnosed positive for SARS-CoV-2 and takes it close to many other unsuspecting users. These users will likely get alerted for exposure risk in spite of no exposure to the actual infected patient. Although it may not be feasible to mitigate such an attack easily, such an attack may not be possible on the large scale, and may not pose a very serious threat; more efficient attacks that do pose serious threats, which might be carried out on a large scale are reviewed in the following discussion.

Replay and Relay Attacks: The proximity identifiers shared or broadcasted by a user who is later diagnosed positive may be misused by malicious entities by replaying them to other users who were not in contact with the infected user. If such identifiers are collected by an adversary (or a colluding group of adversaries) and later replayed to other devices, this is called a *replay attack*. Vaudenay [40] provides an interactive modification of the DP3T protocol that helps in preventing such attacks. A variation of this attack is the *relay attack*, where the identifiers collected from infected users are relayed immediately to other users in different locations, thereby proving the use of timestamps as possible safeguards against replay attacks useless. These attacks are very difficult to prevent. Inclusion of coarse location data as a preventive measure may work out partially—however it could turn out to be a computationally costly solution, and may also compromise users' privacy to a certain extent. In [29], the author provides a novel solution for preventing replay and relay attacks on DP3T through a non-interactive modification.

Inverse Sybil Attacks: *Inverse Sybil attacks*, also called *crown attacks* in [34], are attacks carried out by a computationally strong adversary (e.g. a terrorist group), where many malicious users act as the same user. In (mostly decentralized) contact tracing systems where users send their broadcasted identifiers to the central server on positive diagnosis, multiple malicious users could broadcast the same identifiers to different people at different locations, causing all the receiving users to be falsely alerted of exposure if even one of them reports as a positive case to the server. In (mostly centralized) contact tracing systems where users report the received identifiers to the server on being infected, it is even easier to carry out this attack as it is sufficient for the adversaries to merely broadcast the same identifiers to a large population of users. Protocols that employ interactive exchange of proximity identifiers instead of allowing solely for broadcast are comparatively better protected from such attacks, while potentially incurring other costs (like loss of privacy, false negatives, etc.).

2.2.3 Privacy Attacks

Loss of privacy is another issue that needs to be considered when designing contact tracing systems, particularly when mitigating integrity risks. Inclusion of too many meta-data (e.g. a user's time, coarse location, postal code etc.) may result in a partial loss of privacy or even complete identification. Preventing such loss of privacy is also important for encouraging a large-scale adoption through voluntary usage of the system by citizens without any fear of state surveillance.

Linkage/Deanonymization Attacks: A malicious adversary may monitor communication channels (and an honest entity may also receive some communication data), which may allow for identification (deanonymization) of the communicating users. Secure communication channels, and algorithms with strong privacy should be employed in order to avoid such *linkage attacks*.

Single-entry Attacks: The single-entry attack is a special type of the deanonymization attack, in which a malicious user keeps one's device near the device of another user (without physically coming in proximity) and switching off the device otherwise. In case the malicious user's app declares the user at-risk, it would lead to a conclusion that the targeted user is infected.

This attack may also result in the inadvertent deanonymization of a user if that is coincidentally the only user with whom a person has come into contact over a particular period of time, and has received an exposure alert.

2.2.4 Non-cryptographic Attacks

False Negatives: False negatives may usually occur due to discrepancies in the system such as failure to detect some devices, distorted communication between various entities (user-to-server, health authority-to-server, server-to-user, etc.), inaccurate computation of exposure score, etc. These issues are mostly non-cryptographic and unavoidable to some extent.

Denial of Service (DoS): Denial of service, especially by the central server (and possibly health authority) could occur because of factors like a high volume of communication, which may cause a drain on the storage capacity or even the power of the server, defective or incompatible settings in the device, bluetooth or other software, etc. Measures such as use of less costly algorithms may help in reducing these faults.

We now look into the details of some centralized systems that are already in use in some countries. We also analyze a few protocols that are actively being considered for implementation in some other countries.

2.3 BlueTrace, OpenTrace and TraceTogether

2.3.1 Framework

BlueTrace [8, 10] is an open source application layer protocol developed by the Singapore Government Digital Services for digital contact tracing systems. Open-Trace [5] is a reference implementation of the BlueTrace protocol under the GPL-3.0 license, which includes the generic code-base for the app (Android and iOS) as well as for the server. TraceTogether [37] is a specific implementation of OpenTrace that is being used by the Singapore Government for digital contact tracing and it supports the efforts of the Ministry of Health's contact tracers. In this section, we primarily focus on the framework of BlueTrace protocol as it constitutes the basic layer on top of which the reference implementation and the apps are built.

2.3.2 Design Principles

A stated design principle of BlueTrace is that it is "designed around privacy" [8, 10]. The principle has been elaborated using the following salient points.

1. The BlueTrace peer-to-peer messages contain temporary identifiers that change frequently. So a third party (i.e., a party other than the app that sends the message and the central server) sniffing such messages, would be unable to identify the device or track the movement of the registered user.
2. The only personally-identifiable data point required by the protocol is the user's phone number. The number is securely stored in the central server by the health authority.
3. The protocol stores the proximity information (or the encounter history) locally in each user's device as collected through the peer-to-peer messages. This encounter history stored within a device is shared with the central server only when (a) the user is found to be infected and (b) the user chooses to share it.
4. A user can decide to revoke one's consent of usage of the app at any point of time. As soon as the user withdraws consent, the server deletes all personally identifiable or link-able information about the user. Hence, encounter history from other installed apps can no longer be linked to this user.

The other core design principle of BlueTrace is that it is built around the supervision of the health authority. This is implied in the following ways.

1. The central server is expected to be administered by a trusted health authority as it is responsible for registering the user through personally identifiable information (phone number, etc.).
2. The temporary identifiers are generated and supplied to the apps by the central server.

3. The encounter history of the infected user is uploaded to the central server which
   then finds out the possible primary contacts by matching the encounter history
   with registered users' database and helps the health authority to notify the corresponding users.
4. A federated system of central servers administered by multiple health authorities
   (in multiple countries/regions/jurisdictions) can communicate among each other
   to identify and notify possible primary contacts who may have traveled across
   countries/regions/jurisdictions.

It must be noted that although we have placed BlueTrace under centralized digital
contact tracing systems, the documentation of BlueTrace considers its architecture
to have both centralized and decentralized components where the decentralization
aspect comes from the way peer-to-peer messages are passed and the encounter
history is stored in the devices.

2.3.3 Protocol Details

The following sequence diagram (Fig. 2.1) can be used to describe the BlueTrace
protocol.

There are three entities in this diagram—(a) the reporting server (b) the client
(central) and (c) the client (peripheral). The *reporting server* is the same as what we
have referred to as the central server so far. The *client (central)* and *client (peripheral)* can be viewed as two apps or two users communicating through peer-to-peer
messages built on top of BLE (Bluetooth Low Energy), where one party plays the
role of *central* by scanning for presence of other devices, while the other plays the
role of *peripheral* by advertising its presence. When a *central* discovers a *peripheral*,
it records the peripheral's packet and sends its own packet to the peripheral. Each
device plays the role of central vs peripheral in a 1 : 4 ratio of time-slices in a duty
cycle. However, there could be some devices that always remain in the peripheral
state. The communication that we have described just now falls under Device-to-
Device Communication Protocol (DDC) part of BlueTrace, which we describe next.

2.3.3.1 Device-to-Device Communication Protocol (DDC)

These messages are created using UTF-8 encoded JSON data interchange format and
include the information about temporary ID, device model, signal strength (when
operating as a central), Health Authority Identifier (HAI) and BlueTrace protocol
version. These messages are sent in an unencrypted fashion. The signal strength is
coded using Received Signal Strength Indication (RSSI) format. Since temporary
IDs are not link-able to the users of the devices and these IDs are constantly rotated,
there is seemingly no immediate security or privacy risk of this disclosure even in
the presence of malicious apps or software listening to such packets.

Fig. 2.1 Description of
BlueTrace

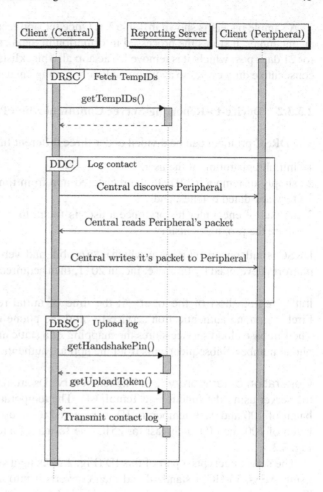

Table 2.1 A sample packet

{
    "id": "FmFISm9nq3PgpLdxxYpTx5tF3ML3Va1wqqgY9DGDz1utPbw+Iz8tqAdpbxR1 nSvr+ILXPG==", // TempID

    "md": "iPhone X", // Device model

    "rc": −60, // Signal strength

    "o": "IJ_HAI", // Health authority identifier

    "v": 2 // Protocol version

}

A sample packet is shown in Table 2.1. Once the app receives such a packet from an encounter, it stores the processed information in the local database of the device for 21 days post which, it is removed. The app also blacklists the other device for two consecutive duty cycles to avoid immediately getting engaged with the same device.

2.3.3.2 Device-to-Reporting-Server Communication Protocol (DRSC)

The DRSC protocol can be divided under three different functions:

1. initial registration of the user,
2. supply of temporary IDs to the registered app from time to time in the form of forward-dated batches, and
3. upload of encounter history once a user is found to be infected and chooses to share the proximity history.

DRSC is built on top of Firebase, which is "a mobile and web application development platform developed by Firebase, Inc. in 2011, then acquired by Google in 2014" [9].

Initial registration of the user: At the time of initial registration, the app uses Firebase phone authentication service to bind the phone number with the device. The Firebase cloud service stores the mapping of a static and unique user ID to that phone number. Subsequent calls from the app are authenticated using this ID.

Generation of temporary IDs: The temporary IDs are requested by the app from the server using the function getTempIDs(). The temporary IDs are generated in a batch of 100 and each temporary ID is expected to be used for 15 min implying a batch of 100 such IDs may last for 25 h. The format of a temporary ID is shown in Fig. 2.2.
The server encrypts a part of this ID (Fig. 2.2) using a symmetric encryption key using AES-256-GCM standard and then converts it into a Base64 encoded string. The secret key of the symmetric encryption is known only to the server and hence that part of the ID can neither be deciphered nor tampered by any other party. The IV part of the ID is generated using a PRNG (Pseudo-Random-Number-Generator) algorithm and the Auth Tag is used for integrity check.

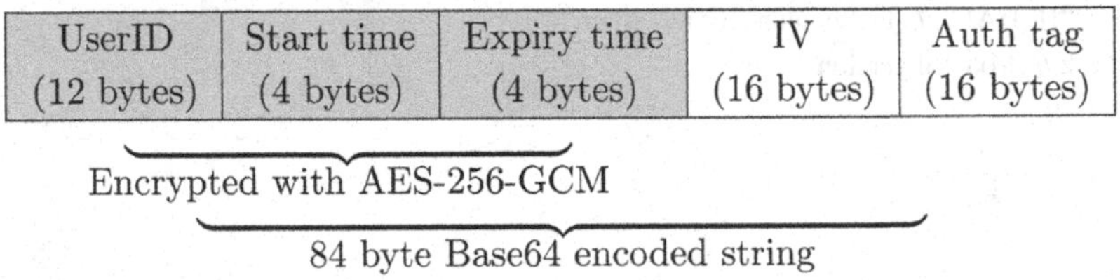

UserID (12 bytes)	Start time (4 bytes)	Expiry time (4 bytes)	IV (16 bytes)	Auth tag (16 bytes)

Encrypted with AES-256-GCM

84 byte Base64 encoded string

Fig. 2.2 Format of temporary ID

Upload of encounter history: The upload of the encounter history starts with the invocation of function getHandshakePin() to obtain an authenticated PIN for uploading the data to the cloud server. Next, getUploadToken() function is called to get a single-use token for the upload. A JSON file is created with the upload token and the encounter history of the last 21 days by using the writeToInternalStorageAnd Upload() function. Finally, the file is uploaded to the Google cloud using uploadTo-CloudStorage() function. There is no separate encryption applied to this file at the time of upload and the stored file's security is based on the settings of Google Cloud Storage encryption.

2.3.3.3 Contact Tracing at the Server End

Once the encounter history is uploaded by an infected user's app, the server analyzes each of the packets to check if the HAI (Health Authority Identification) within the packet belongs to its own jurisdiction or some other Health Authority.

If the HAI corresponds to its own jurisdiction, it inspects the packets and decrypts the temporary ID using the symmetric secret key to detect if the encounter time-stamps are within the valid duration (based on the *start time* and *expiry time* marked inside the packet) of the messages. It ignores a packet if it is not within the valid duration—this prevents the possible replay attacks on the protocol. For valid packets, it retrieves the relevant information like the signal strengths and correlates multiple packets to decide the duration of the encounter with any specific user. Epidemio-logical parameters (like the duration of contact and the proximity based on signal strength) are used to decide if the user from whose device a set of messages were received by the infected user, can be considered a *close contact* or not. If the encounter is indeed considered a close contact (close encounter), the phone number is retrieved based on the user ID contained within the packets. The contact tracing team of the health authority would then reach out to the relevant user associated with the phone number and continue the contact tracing process as followed in the manual version of contact tracing. The OpenTrace implementation has not automated this step of notification and has let it remain a human-centric and human-led process.

2.3.3.4 Server-to-Server Communication Protocol

If the HAI belongs to a different health authority, the server (belonging to health authority A in Fig. 2.3) passes the encrypted temporary IDs to that server under health authority B, so that the server B may decrypt the same by referring to its data-store B to identify the relevant user ID and returns a PseudoID (*salted cryptographic hash*) of the user ID back to server A. Server A uses such PseudoIDs to identify the possible close encounters and notifies the PseudoIDs that can be considered close contacts back to health authority server B.

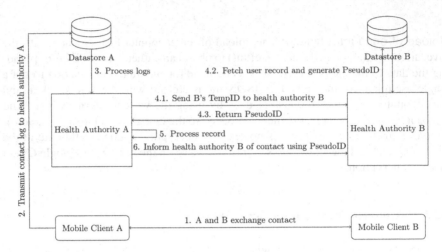

Fig. 2.3 Server to server communication

2.3.4 Highlights and Characteristics

We now look at some of the highlights and characteristics of the proposal.

- **"Human-in-the-loop" system:** BlueTrace has been designed as a protocol to extend the manual contact tracing process of a Government or health authority by decentralized automated recall of contacts through a digital contact tracing system while maintaining the contact tracing of probable close contacts of infected individuals centralized under the supervision of the Government's or health authority's contact tracing team.
- **Minimal collection of personally identifiable data:** Apart from phone numbers, no other personally identifiable data of the users get stored/tracked in the system.
- **A user's identity is stored only in the data-store of the health authority to which the user belongs:** Neither the device to device communication nor the server to server communication reveals the static user ID or phone number of a user.
- **Encounter history tracks *who* has been in contact with but not *where*:** The protocol does not require any access to the location of a user's device at any point of time. So, GPS or any other location information (like WiFi scanning) is neither checked nor stored by the protocol.
- **Data upload happens in presence of a contact tracer (for TraceTogether):** The authentication mechanism (of BlueTrace protocol) and the process in place for TraceTogether app, together ensure that the encounter history upload step can happen only in presence of a genuine contact tracer.
- **Configurability and extensibility:** There are many parameters of the protocol that are configurable. For example, the number of days for which the encounter history is stored in a device can be modified as per epidemiologic need. In the current OpenTrace implementation and for TraceTogether it is kept as 21 days.

Similarly, the Bluetooth signal strength (RSSI readings) is used as a proxy for the distance between two devices. In TraceTogether, the actual implementation has been done after doing a careful calibration of various mobile devices from different manufacturers and models as used in Singapore. This calibration data is provided as a baseline dataset and any implementation of BlueTrace protocol can potentially refine it as per the need in a different country / region. Similarly, the final step of alerting users about possible contact event(s) can also be automated by implementing additional notification APIs between a device and the server. Implementations of BlueTrace under separate health authorities can also modify the ratio of scanning and advertising periods within a duty cycle. Similarly, the algorithm for generating Temp IDs and PseudoIDs can be tweaked as per need of the health authority.

- **BlueTrace uses BLE in Connected Topology mode:** Bluetooth enabled devices can communicate through BLE in two modes [36]—broadcast topology mode and connected topology mode. In the broadcast topology mode, a broadcasting device can simultaneously broadcast messages to multiple observers. However, the BlueTrace designers opted for the connected topology mode in which a device while playing the role of a central needs to establish connection with another peripheral device before exchanging BLE packets between each other.

2.3.5 System Analysis

This section provides analyses of the protocols from different aspects.

2.3.5.1 Security and Privacy Analysis

The security and privacy of BlueTrace protocol hinges upon two key design elements:

1. the centralized symmetric key encryption (and decryption) at the server-end of temporary identifiers and
2. the decentralized logging of such IDs during the encounter of two devices.

The encounter history of a user remains unknown and hence private from the health authority unless the user is tested SARS-CoV-2 positive. The identity of a user (whether infected or not) remains unknown and private to any other user and any other authority. The location information is unknown to any entity and hence the protocol cannot be used on its own to track any user. The personally identifiable information (static unique user ID and phone number of the user) are stored in the central data store. The security of any such data depends upon the security scheme adopted between the central server and central data store and the symmetric key encryption used in the DRSC protocol. There is no separate encryption scheme used in BLE packets; the local data storage does not include any additional security or privacy considerations other than what is guaranteed by Android or iOS apps in their respective operating environments.

Cryptographic Primitives and Encodings Used

- **AES-256-GCM.** AES-256-GCM is the 256-bit keyed initialization of the *Authenticated Encryption Standard* that uses the *Galois Counter Mode*. This mode of operation is capable of authenticated encryption of a message as well as verifying the integrity and authenticity of of additional authenticated data, and is specified in the NIST Special Publication 800-38D [22].
- **Base64 encoding.** In order to avoid corruption of data during transmission due to reasons such as interpreting binary data as text, control characters, etc., it is encoded before sending over any channel. One such method of encoding is the base64 encoding, which is a binary-to text encoding scheme that translates the input into a *radix*-64 representation (every 6 bits of the input message is encoded into a 64-bit code).
- **IV generation.** The term IV stands for *initialization vector* (also *starting vector*). As its name suggests, it is a fixed-length input provided at the initiation of of cryptographic implementation. The main purpose of this input is to provide randomization to the implemented scheme or construction, and is generated through a *pseudorandom permutation* so as to satisfy the requirement of uniqueness—no IV must repeat under the same key.
- **Authentication tag.** An authentication tag or a *Message Authentication Code* (MAC) is a cryptographic scheme of message authentication. An authentication tag is used to prevent *forgery* of messages; it maintains the authenticity of the message (i.e. the message was truly sent by the sender as claimed) as well as its integrity (i.e. the message received is unchanged and the same as the message sent), when sent over a communication channel.
- **Salted cryptographic hash.** A salt is a random value input to a cryptographic scheme, usually to passwords before hashing, implementing one-way functions, etc. It is similar to an IV, but holds an important distinction with it in that it may be repeated, as it is generated by a *pseudorandom function*.

Protection Against Security Attacks

- **Backend impersonation.** Since the backend server for any implementation is expected to have a well-known domain name with proper certification, the scope of a backend impersonation attack is limited. However, if the communication channel between the app and the server is secure and authenticated, the system would be more robust against such attacks.
- **Server-end data breach.** The protocol can be subjected to such an attack since the server is the nerve center in the framework of this protocol and stores personally identifiable data.
- **Replay attack.** The chance of such an attack is limited to within 15 min at maximum as the temporary IDs expire after that time.
- **Relay attack.** BlueTrace is susceptible to relay attack.

- **Deanonymization.** This is not possible from device end alone without additional contextual data (like side channel attack). However, if the server data is compromised, the user data may easily get deanonymized.
- **Coercion threats.** User-end devices do not store any personally identifiable information, and hence the extent of damage through coercion threats would be limited. However, if the device of an infected user is in the possession of a malicious third party, there is a significant chance of it being misused to create a large number of false positives in the system.
- **Other attacks.** BlueTrace cannot be subjected to the inverse-Sybil attack as multiple devices cannot impersonate the same user. One-entry attack is also possible in BlueTrace, OpenTrace and TraceTogether; the extent of damage through such an attack on these protocols would be limited since the alerting mechanism is a human contact tracer-led process.

It is important to keep in mind the possible open areas. Based on this analysis, it may be inferred that server-end data breach is probably the most significant risk in BlueTrace. Apart from that, backend impersonation, deanonymization and relay attacks may also need to be handled by putting some counter-measures in place.

2.3.5.2 Architecture Analysis

Use of the BLE connected topology mode: While this topology provides the advantage of symmetric communication of encounter messages between two devices in proximity, the downside is that it is not as "easy or fast to use" [36] as compared to the broadcast topology. The additional advantage of encrypting the packets in connected topology mode has not been utilized in BlueTrace.

Upload of encounter data by the infected user's app: The advantage of this scheme is the optimization of data upload since only data that need to be shared with the health authority is uploaded and all other encounter history remains private; the disadvantage is that the infected user's device can become the single-point-of failure. If the device crashes or the local data becomes corrupted/inaccessible for some reason, the entire contact history would be lost.

Centralized security of sensitive and personally identifiable data: This ensures that if the centralized storage mechanism is made robust and secure (at the equivalent level of any sensitive Government data), the possibility of it getting compromised would be remote. At the same time, such a centralized store is subject to single-point-failure and dependent upon the safety and security mechanisms implemented by private entities like Google or Apple. As pointed out by Robert Valk in his article [38], for OpenTrace implementation, Google Cloud Services "stores your data, manages the encryption keys, links the mobile number and unique ID of every user, executes the server-less functions, provides the cryptographic libraries as part of the cloud function's runtime, and controls the Android app distribution channels."

Challenge faced by iOS users: This is an important issue to be considered as a possible open area. Apple restricts the usage of the connected topology mode of BLE by not allowing it to run in the background in iOS. Due to this, iPhone users need to run TraceTogether in the foreground. This creates inconvenience. TraceTogether team has mentioned in an article [17], "To help users keep the app running in the foreground while minimizing battery usage, the TraceTogether team included a power saver mode setting in the code-base. If you are an iPhone user, all you have to do is keep TraceTogether open but place the phone upside down in your pocket or face down on the table. That will trigger the power saver mode, allowing the app to regularly scan the environment for other TraceTogether users."

2.4 COVIDSafe

2.4.1 Framework

COVIDSafe [13] is the official digital contact tracing app released by the Australian Government on 26 April, 2020 and is based on the BlueTrace protocol designed and developed by the Singapore Government Digital Services. The code-base for both the Android and the iOS systems have been released as open source repositories in github [6, 7].

In this section, we primarily describe the app-specific customizations and changes adopted at the implementation stage that are not a standard part of the BlueTrace protocol. For all other aspects (especially for highlights, characteristics and system analysis) we refer to the sections on BlueTrace, OpenTrace and TraceTogether.

2.4.2 Design Principles

The stated design principle of BlueTrace of "designed around privacy" [8, 10] continues to be emphasized in the case of COVIDSafe. The privacy policy has been well-documented [30] and an extensive Privacy Impact Assessment Report [14] as well as the Department of Health's response to it have been made public. All the design principles of BlueTrace apply to the implementation of COVIDSafe except the following-

1. There are quite a few personally-identifiable data points captured by the app at the time of initial registration. These are-

   - **Mobile phone number.** This is used later for contacting the individuals who are identified by the system as "at-risk of being infected".

- **Name.** This is mentioned later to ensure that the right individual is contacted by the health officials from the State or the Territory. If uncomfortable sharing one's real name, a user is free to mention any "pseudonym or fake name".
- **Age range.** This data point is used by health officials to decide on the prioritization of who should be contacted with urgency.
- **Postcode.** This data point allows the health department to assign the appropriate health official from the designated state or territory corresponding to that post code to contact the individuals and decide on which area to be declared as hotspot etc.

2. If a user decides to delete the app and discontinue its usage, the website provides the following information [13]-
"You can delete the COVIDSafe app from your phone at any time. This will delete all COVIDSafe app information from your phone. The information in the secure information storage system will not be deleted immediately. It will be destroyed at the end of the pandemic. If you would like your information deleted from the storage system sooner, you can complete our request data deletion form."

One may have a look at [14, 41] for privacy and legislative issues in this regard.

2.4.3 Protocol Implementation Details

There are not many differences in the implementation of the protocol as compared to what has already been described under OpenTrace and TraceTogether, except the following-

- The backend of COVIDSafe runs on the Amazon Web Services (AWS) platform (not on Google Cloud) and the server data is stored in AWS Sydney region data center so that the Australian Government may have the legal jurisdiction over the data center.
- A user wanting to change one's registration information may do so by deleting the app and reinstalling it with the desired changes. A user may also modify information such as one's name, age-range and postcode with uninstall-reinstallation process, but not the phone number. A user may also contact the Department of Health and submit a relevant form to delete all of one's data from the system.
- The encrypted user ID is the basis on which the "de-identified reports about uptake of COVIDSafe" and "analytical data from iTunes and Google Play about COVID-Safe including the number of downloads, average use time and deletions" would be collected by Digital Transformation Agency of Government of Australia.
- Certain bugs [32] that originally got detected and then fixed in OpenTrace, re-appeared in the COVIDSafe implementation; these were eventually rectified in a subsequent release (13 May, 2020).
- Currently, the implementation does not allow any user to register using a phone number other than that from Australia (with country code of +61).

2.4.4 Highlights, Characteristics and System Analysis

The highlights, characteristics and system analyses for COVIDSafe being almost identical to those in the corresponding subsections of BlueTrace, shall not be mentioned separately. However, there are certain differences for the following functionalities-

- **Personally identifiable data.** Apart from phone numbers, a few other personally identifiable information that is collected by the app includes the name, postcode and age-range. However, it is allowed to share a pseudonym or a fake name in place of the actual name of the user.
- **Data upload process for a user tested positive.** Once a user chooses to upload the contact details captured by one's app over the last 21 days, a health official initiates the authentication process. As part of the authentication mechanism, the health official sends a PIN number (through the system) to the user's registered phone number (over SMS) so that the person may use that to upload the relevant contact information from the device to the backend server.

2.5 Centralized Systems with Private Specifications

The following systems and protocols have user-level documentation and in some cases client-side source code in the public domain; detailed technical specifications have not been explained in details in certain cases. We have already given an outline of the Aarogya Setu app in the previous chapter. We add a few more details in this section.

Aarogya Setu: At the time of initial registration, Aarogya Setu asks for the user's mobile number, name, gender, profession, age and the list of countries visited in the last 30 days. In addition, it also requests the user to mention if he/she is willing to volunteer in the times of need. The information collected from the user at the time of registration is securely stored in the central server. The server also generates a unique pseudorandom Device iDentity (DiD) number for each user and associates the same with the encrypted personally identifiable set of information at the backend database. For all subsequent communications between the devices coming in proximity with each other or between the device and the server, this DiD is used. At the time of recording the contact events, a user app also records the (time, duration, location and distance) corresponding to each nearby device's app (in addition to the unique randomized identifier shared by that device).

All the local device data gets encrypted using Advanced Encryption Standards (AES) before storing. Any device data that is older than 14 days gets automatically deleted. Similarly, the longest period for which the user data remains undisturbed at the server end is 60 days.

Whenever the user takes a self-assessment, that data along with the location of the user gets transferred and securely stored in the backend server. Whenever a person is tested positive, that data from the Indian Council of Medical Research (ICMR) is shared with the Aarogya Setu server. If the infected user has the Aarogya Setu app installed, then a notification is sent to the user-app for changing the color to "Red", the proximity data captured by that person's device would be uploaded to the server so that the contact tracing process can be started by identifying the individuals who might be at-risk based on their exposures. Individual user-apps also calculate the risk status by communicating with the server to discover if the owner was in proximity with any known infected user or not. It has been mentioned in the FAQ document that Aarogya Setu collects a user's location for two purposes, namely-

1. to identify the possible hot-spots where infections could be spreading and
2. to understand the routes traversed by the infected individuals so that appropriate measures like sanitization and isolation of affected individuals may be implemented easily.

PEPP-PT NTK: The Pan-European Privacy-Preserving Proximity Tracing Need-To-Know System [1] has been designed jointly by a number of European institutes and organizations, including the Fraunhofer Institute for Telecommunications, Robert Koch Institute, Technical University of Berlin, TU Dresden, University of Erfurt and Vodafone Germany.

In this protocol, the temporary IDs that are shared by a device as proximity IDs have a mapping with the user's persistent ID. This mapping is maintained at the server end. When a user is diagnosed positive, all the received temporary IDs from his/her device get uploaded to the server. The server decrypts the temporary IDs to identify the persistent IDs of the users who have significant risks and notifies them through a push or pull mechanism. The risk computation depends on the number of contacts of a user with the infected users and the durations and distances (as decoded from the signal strengths of the received signals) between the devices in each such contact event.

As per current information [44], it appears that only Georgia has implemented this protocol in their Stop Covid contact tracing system.

NHS_COVID-19: The NHS_COVID-19 app had received significant attention before the UK Government decided to abandon the initiative [24] in favor of the Exposure Notification APIs jointly developed by Apple and Google. The main reason behind this decision [42] appears to be the experience from the pilot roll-out, in which the app was able to detect only 4% of the iPhone devices and 75% of the Android based mobile phones, whereas Google/Apple system could catch 99% of the devices.

Released with the free-ware licensing scheme in the United Kingdom on 6 May, 2020, this app was developed by NHSX with the help of VMWare and a team of scientists and doctors, and launched as a pilot test release in the Isle of Wight. The client-side code-base for both the Android and the iOS systems were released as open source repositories in github [26, 27].

We outline some characteristics of this protocol, particularly as it may be reasonable to expect that the new app being developed using Google/Apple APIs may retain some of these features.

- An interesting differences of this app from other apps was that it allowed a user to notify NHS in case he/she felt unwell (to some extent this is similar to the self-assessment option of Aarogya Setu), which in turn could trigger alerts from NHS to other users of the app who might have come in close contact of this user in the past 28 days.
- The *contact risk model* developed by NHS was being constantly updated to enhance its accuracy.
- No personally identifiable data was collected by the app. However, the anonymized data sets were planned to "be used for NHS care, management, evaluation and research". The types of data collected by the app included (a) first half of the postal code of the user's area and (b) the make and model of the mobile device.
- Users were allowed to delete the app whenever they wanted and the NHS was committed to follow the data regulations for the usage of the anonymized data.
- The app did not collect any location information.
- Certain questions [31] were raised about the possible security and privacy issues of the collected data and usability challenges (like the requirement of keeping the app in the foreground).

2.6 ROBERT and DESIRE: Centralized to Decentralized

Considering the overall framework, ROBERT and DESIRE both have the essence of decentralized as well as centralized systems. The ROBust and privacy-presERving proximity Tracing (ROBERT) [19, 20] scheme is a digital contact tracing protocol specification that has jointly been designed by the PRIVATICS project team from Inria, France and Fraunhofer, AISEC, Germany under the aegis of the Pan-European Privacy-Preserving Proximity Tracing (PEPP-PT/PEPP) initiative [28]. DESIRE [12] has been proposed as an evolution of the ROBERT protocol by the PRIVATICS project team from Inria, France. Both ROBERT and DESIRE have been designed with the intent of bringing the best of centralized and decentralized systems. Hence, it can be placed right in the middle of these two approaches. Precisely for that reason, we position the description of this pair of protocols at the end of the chapter on centralized schemes before we venture into the decentralized digital contact tracing systems.

In each of the following subsections we first describe the ROBERT protocol and then present the changes that have been incorporated in the DESIRE proposal.

2.6.1 Design Principles

The security and privacy requirements and the design goals for ROBERT and DESIRE are stated in the respective specification documents [12, 20]. However, the design principles are not separately articulated. In our view, there are three prominent design principles that can be interpreted from the specifications, which stand out as the guiding factors behind the design decisions. These are as follows.

1. **Hybrid approach.** The first design principle is that centralized as well as decentralized features must be judiciously combined in a digital contact tracing system instead of creating either a fully centralized framework, which may compromise on privacy requirements or a fully decentralized framework, which may compromise on security and robustness requirements. This is evident from the statement in the abstract of the ROBERT specification that mentions, "Although it might seem attractive in terms of privacy to adopt a fully decentralized solution, such approaches face inherent challenges in terms of security and robustness against malicious users" [20].

2. **Adaptable design.** The second design principle that can be interpreted from the specifications is that the protocols propose to construct the framework in the form of configurable components in such a way that the entire system can be adapted towards a fully centralized or a fully decentralized system. We shall elaborate more on this principle when we describe the details of the DESIRE protocol in this section.

3. **Generalized adversarial model:** ROBERT assumes the threat of malicious users and an *honest-but-curious* authority (server) against whose attacks the protocol needs to be robust whereas DESIRE considers the adversarial model to be a fully generalized one in presence of malicious users, malicious authorities and a collusion of both the parties.

Some of the design goals of ROBERT are subjective (or loosely defined) in nature while the rest are specific and verifiable. The subjective goals are:

- The system must be simple to understand and use.
- It must be transparent.
- It should be possible to deploy the system with minimal infrastructure.

The specific goals that can be verified in any implementation are:

- **Maintenance of anonymity.** Neither the client app side nor the server side of the protocol may collect or store any personal (or personally identifiable) data.
- **Federated infrastructure.** The system is expected to scale beyond one country or region and the server side architecture and primitives are designed assuming that the multiple trusted authorities can manage the different servers that would communicate and cooperate with each other.

These design goals are not separately listed down in the DESIRE specification. We may however assume that all these design goals are also valid for DESIRE, consid-

ering that it is an extension of the ROBERT protocol (except the federated infrastructure, since the protocol, rather surprisingly, has not retained any such provision).

Apart from the above design goals, the security and privacy requirements are as
follows:

- The proximity data must be accurate and reliable. This is a subjective requirement
  and is not quantified in the specification so as to derive the extent to which false
  positives or false negatives can be tolerated.
- No user or central authority (in general) should be able to identify in real-time or
  discover through post-processing, the identity of another user (whether infected
  or not). Similarly, no such party should be able to detect the location of another
  user or reconstruct a social graph around another person.

2.6.2 Protocol Details

Both ROBERT and DESIRE are designed to use BLE in broadcast topology mode
and not in the connected topology mode. DESIRE is more explicit in its description
of packet structure and the mechanism of using the broadcast topology, but the
specification for ROBERT does not elaborate the BLE. Hence, at the lowest level
of the protocol stack, they are expected to behave differently from BlueTrace. The
pros and cons of this choice has not been discussed in the specification. The efficacy
of this choice can be analyzed only when a reference implementation is tested or an
actual implementation of ROBERT (or DESIRE) is rolled out for any country. We
first focus on ROBERT in depth and then describe the ways in which DESIRE differs
from ROBERT by explaining the new primitives, processes and functionalities.

A device running an app based on ROBERT broadcasts HELLO messages through
BLE, which other nearby devices can capture and store. Similarly, it simultaneously
captures HELLO messages broadcasted by other devices.

2.6.2.1 Structure and Usage of the HELLO Message

The HELLO message is 128-bit long and consists of four parts:

- ECC: Encrypted Country Code (8-bits)—described in detail below.
- EBID: Ephemeral Bluetooth IDentifier (64-bits)—described in detail below.
- Time: 16-bit truncated (less-significant-bits) part of the current time-stamp incor-
  porated to prevent replay attacks.
- MAC: Message Authentication Code (40 bits) and is intended to prevent integrity
  attacks.

The most important part is the Ephemeral Bluetooth IDentifier (EBID). Within the
context of digital contact tracing Systems, the term 'ephemeral' has been used for
the first time in case of DP-3T protocol. As the term suggests, these IDs are meant to

be short-lived. It serves the purpose of being a pseudorandom number corresponding to an instance of the app and for a specific time-interval. EBIDs change at regular intervals. This number is designed to not reveal any personally identifiable user information. Its value constantly changes in a random fashion—hence, no one can possibly track a user from a series of these numbers emitted by the app installed in the user's device. However, these numbers would eventually play a crucial role in the identification of proximity events from which the ROBERT protocol-based system can deduce whether a user might have been infected or not.

Let us now understand how an EBID is constructed and used. EBID is derived as

$$EBID = ENC(K_{Server}, i \mid ID_A).$$

Here, ENC stands for an encryption algorithm and as per the protocol specification it is expected to be implemented as a 64-bit block cipher like SKINNY-64/192 [9].

The parameters K_{Server}, i and ID_A are used as a key to the algorithm. ID_A is a permanent identifier attached to user A and is known only to the server to which the app registers initially at the time of installation. The integer i stands for an epoch number (achieved by discretization of time-intervals) and EBID value remains unchanged for an epoch typically of a duration of 15 min as per the recommendations of the Bluetooth specifications [11].

K_{Server} is an L-bit long server key ($L \geq 128$) known only to the server. From this description, it is evident that only the server can create this identifier and the app on its own can neither create it nor decrypt any of its parameters including the permanent identifier ID_A. ENC^{-1} is the inverse of ENC, which means it is the decryption algorithm using which the server can retrieve back ID_A and the epoch number i from EBID using the server key K_{Server}.

Encrypted Country Code (ECC) is derived from a publicly known 8-bit Country Code (CC) of the user's country by encrypting it using a federation key K_G, known only to the trusted set of federated servers from the participating European countries and also the EBID value allocated to the user for the corresponding time-interval or epoch (i).

Once an app receives a HELLO message from a nearby device, it first checks if the time value is within a tolerable range of the current system time-stamp (to be precise the truncated version of the system time-stamp) and if the time value is permissible, it stores the entire HELLO message along with the current system time-stamp in its *LocalProximityList*, which is maintained for a certain number of configurable days (e.g. 14 days) and deleted permanently thereafter.

After a regular number of intervals (in terms of epochs), the server, upon explicit request from the app, sends a list of T pairs of (EBID, ECC) where each pair is designated for a specific epoch (i). For all practical purposes, the EBID and ECC values are nothing more than pair of random numbers to the client-side of the app. Whenever the app receives a HELLO message, it can demarcate the positions of the bits corresponding to ECC, EBID, Time and MAC and also verify whether it has been tampered with or not by checking the MAC; however it can not decipher the contents of EBID or ECC. This makes the peer-to-peer messages tamper-proof and secured even in the unsecured broadcast topology mode of BLE (Bluetooth Low Energy) protocol.

The usage of EBIDs in case of a user who is tested positive would be as follows.

2.6.2.2 Exposure Status Reporting

Once a user (say A) is diagnosed as SARS-CoV-2 positive, she may choose to declare the EBIDs her app has captured during the last CT days where CT represents a time-period for which she could have been contagious for others who have come in her close proximity. She would require to get the relevant authorization (e.g. a pre-approved token) from a health authority to upload the (HELLO, Time) pairs from the app's *LocalProximityList*. The exact process of upload authorization has not been elaborated in the specification and we may assume that it could vary from one country to another.

It is interesting to note that during the upload process, A does not reveal any of her EBIDs. Moreover, the specification has recommended that the upload of the entire list of (HELLO, Time) pairs should not be done in a batch mode. In the batch mode of upload, there could be a possibility of a curious authority constructing the social graphs of contact events at the server end. This may eventually lead to re-identification of user identities with the help of circumstantial meta-data for the events. Hence, the specification has suggested that the upload step may use (a) some type of Mixnet or proxy or (b) some trusted intermediate server (like a hospital's server) that would mix the *LocalProximityList*s of multiple users diagnosed as positive and later upload the data to the backend server or (c) have a secured hardware component at the server end that can be accessed only via a set of secured APIs, which can mask any information about the originating apps/devices that had uploaded the lists. We have mentioned earlier that the server can retrieve back the permanent identifier (ID_{User}) of a user and the corresponding epoch number (i) from any one of its EBIDs using the decrypting function $ENC^{-1}(\ldots)$. Hence, after receiving the (HELLO, Time) pairs in the upload process from an app, the server resolves the permanent identifiers for the users that got exposed to A and the corresponding epoch numbers when those users came in close contact with A. The server adds these epoch numbers in a *List of Exposed Epochs (LEE)* maintained in a table (called IDTable) indexed by the permanent identifiers along with some more information about each user's app. Since the server does not store any personally identifiable information (like phone number) against a permanent identifier, it can't (and is not expected to proactively) inform about the exposure event to any user's app. The user's app has to make any explicit request about the exposure status to the server in order to know about its current risk of being infected by the virus.

Next, we describe the process of exposure status detection.

2.6.2.3 Exposure Status Detection

The user-app needs to query the server to know the user's exposure status. In this query (called ESR_REQUEST), the app sends its current set of values comprising EBID, epoch number (i) and time-stamp along with a message authentication code to avoid the possibility of an adversary tampering with the request packet. The server resolves the permanent identifier of the user (ID_{User}) from the EBID and finds out if the LEE list corresponding to ID_{User} is empty or not.

If the list is empty the server responds back with a binary flag bit of 0 (indicating that the user is not at risk). On the other hand, if the list is non-empty, then it uses a publicly known algorithm (as per the guidance of epidemiologists and the health authority) that uses the stored data (primarily from LEE) to identify if the risk probability is above a threshold and if it is above such a threshold, declares the user at risk by returning a bit 1 for the binary flag. At the same time, it marks the UN (User Notified) flag against the permanent identifier as *true* (1). Irrespective of the status (at risk or not at risk), the server updates the SRE (Status Request Epoch) field with the epoch number contained in the ESR_REQUEST as long as the request is a valid one.

An ESR_REQUEST is considered valid if:

- the UN flag was not already set to 1 earlier,
- the request has been received at least after a desired (configurable) minimum number of epochs after the previous request,
- has a correct epoch number,
- has a time-stamp within the tolerable range of current network time, and
- has the correct message authentication code, signifying that there was no tampering with the message.

Once the app receives the *at-risk* flag in ESR_REPLY from the server set to 1, it stops sending any further ESR_REQUEST to the server, notifies an appropriate message at the application level to the user (so that he/she can take the next steps like getting in touch with a health agency for testing etc.) and keeps sending HELLO messages to the nearby devices.

2.6.2.4 Initial Registration

When a user (say A) decides to use an app based on the protocol, she downloads the app from an approved store like Google app store (if her device has Android operating system) or from Apple store (if her device is iOS based) and installs it in her device. At the time of user registration of her app, no personal information of A (like phone number) or device information (like IMEI number or location) is shared with the backend server and the server ensures that she is assigned a permanent identifier (ID_A) in the IDTable maintained at the server-end which remains known only to the server and the user is aware of her unique user-id required for signing in to the app.

Although it has not been mentioned explicitly anywhere in the specification, there seems to be an one-on-one mapping maintained at server end between the user-id (presumably chosen by A) and ID_A.

At the time of registration, the server also keeps a record of additional information for A including (and not limited to) an authentication key (K-Auth$_A$) that would be used to authenticate the messages coming from A's app, an encryption key (K-Enc$_A$) that would be used to encrypt sensitive information to be shared with A's app, UN-flag (User Notification) for A (initially set to *false*), SRE (Status Request Epoch) to store the epoch when A's app would have sent the most recent ESR_REQUEST and LEE (the List of Exposed Epochs) for A which is initially empty. The server also sends an initial list of (EBID, ECC) code pairs that A's app would use for a certain number of epochs before it requests for an additional list of such pairs from the backend server.

2.6.2.5   Risk Scoring Approach

The specification defers the actual description of the risk scoring algorithm to the implementation stage. It mentions that the methodology shall eventually be guided by recommendations from health authorities and epidemiologists. Thus, it may evolve along with the changing nature of the virus or its transmission mechanism at different stages of the pandemic. The designers have argued that the centralization of risk scoring procedure makes the protocol more flexible as compared to decentralized systems since the algorithm can be changed in one place to seamlessly alter the behavior of the rest of the parts including the client side apps. As the backend is expected to be implemented as a secured and a reliable centralized server (under regular auditing for security and privacy by independent regulatory bodies) with a well-known domain name and certification, the entire system is resilient to attacks that may try to tamper the risk scoring mechanism because unlike decentralized systems, the risk evaluation is not done at individual device level in ROBERT (and DESIRE). To influence the risk score of a user's app, either the malicious user needs to expose himself/herself to an infected person or devise ingenious mechanisms to break robust well-known cryptographically secured communication between the app and the server.

At this point, the specification talks about a binary value to be returned to the app in ESR_REPLY message signifying a status of *at-risk* (binary value of 1) or *not at risk* (binary value of 0). The designers have also kept a provision open for returning a probability value instead of a binary value or returning a value of 1 even for a small percentage of users who are not at risk, at random. The latter approach can be used to prevent a *one entry attack*, in which an adversary may plan to place just one entry (of the target victim) in its *LocalProximityList* and hence when its app is declared *at-risk* by the server, the adversary would still not able to identify with certainty whether the target victim is diagnosed positive or not. However, this approach would increase the false positives to a limited extent like 5–10%.

2.6.2.6 Federated System of Servers

The protocol has been designed to be used across countries in Europe where each country can implement its own version of the app following the ROBERT (or DESIRE) framework and each country can have its own backend server. As long as the HELLO messages follow the structure where the first 8 bits contain the Encrypted Country Code (ECC), the federated systems can inter-operate in the following manner:

The specification illustrates a situation where two users, one from Germany (named Uta) and another user from France (called Bernard) happen to come in close proximity of each other and their apps interchange the HELLO messages on a particular epoch (i). If at a later point of time, one of them (say Uta) is diagnosed positive, his app may follow a process (as recommended by the German authorities) to upload the HELLO messages (including the one received from Bernard) upon Uta's consent to the German server. Once the German server decodes (with the help of the Federation Key, K_G) the first 8-bits of the HELLO message sent by Bernard to Uta and realizes that it corresponds to a user's app registered under France, it forwards the corresponding HELLO message to the France's server. Eventually, the server in France adds a record in the LEE corresponding to Bernard's permanent identifier ($ID_{Bernard}$) about the exposure epoch (i), which can be used during the risk score computation for Bernard.

2.6.3 Protocol Details: Differences in DESIRE

We now describe the specific differences in DESIRE protocol vis-a-vis the ROBERT protocol.

2.6.3.1 Private Encounter Tokens (PETs)

DESIRE proposes the storage of Private Encounter Tokens (PETs) by the devices instead of storing the received EBIDs. The PETs are generated in the following manner:

Suppose A and B happen to come in close proximity to each other. Both A's app and B's app independently generate pseudorandom numbers that remain constant for the duration of an epoch. For example, if A's app has generated a pseudorandom number x (which is only known to A and hence a secret key), it shares the computed value of g^x (public key) as the EBID to the nearby devices including B's device. Let us assume on the other hand B's device generates a pseudorandom number y and shares the computed value of g^y as the EBID to A.

Next, each of the apps records a computed hash value of the EBID received to the power of its own secret as the PET token from the given encounter. Hence, for both the devices this event gets recorded as the same value $H(g^{x \cdot y})$ where H is a cryptographic hash function such as SHA-256. The DESIRE specification also refers to the optional storage of additional metadata like speed, signal strength etc.

From the cryptographic point of view, it has been assumed that both the apps follow the discrete logarithm of elliptic curve (Curve25519) with the same group structure of order p and generator g. In fact, this is the basic idea of Diffie-Hellman key exchange protocol. While this protocol is secure in classical computational model under some usual assumptions, this is absolutely insecure in quantum computational paradigm. Fortunately, commercial quantum computers are still elusive and there are several protocols which are secure in the quantum model too.

At a later point of time, if B happens to be diagnosed SARS-CoV-2 positive, then upon his consent and health authority's requisite approval, all the PET tokens stored in B's device for the last CT days get uploaded to the backend server which adds these to a global *EList*, containing the exposed list of PETs. Sometime later, A enquires the server to know her risk status and at the time of sending the query also uploads the PETs received from other devices (including those that were sent by B's device) in the last 24 h. The server finds a match of the list of exposed PETs as uploaded by B with some PETs uploaded by A. The server then maintains a record of this encounter by adding the epoch numbers and other details corresponding to the encounter in a *List of Exposed PET Metadata* (LEPM) against the permanent ID of A. The server also computes the risk score based on the configured risk scoring algorithm depending upon how many of A's LEPM entries appear in the global *EList* and returns the flag *at-risk* (if the risk threshold has been crossed) or (otherwise) *not-at-risk* to A's app.

The actual implementation of PET tokens, as proposed in the specification of DESIRE, is slightly more complex than what has been described above. It suggests that a device maintains two lists simultaneously where one is called the ETL (Exposure Token List) and the other is called the RTL (Request Token List). For every encounter and computed value of $g^{x \cdot y}$, it stores two PET values $H(``1''|g^{x \cdot y})$ and $H(``2''|g^{x \cdot y})$ in such a way that the PET value that gets stored in A's device in ETL is the same as the PET value that gets stored in B's device in RTL and vice-versa. B, once diagnosed positive, uploads the PET values from its ETL while A uses the PET values contained in her device's RTL while sending the ESR_REQUEST message to the backend server. This has been done so that a curious server would not be able to build a social graph for any infected user as the uploaded PET tokens of B that his app uploads after him being diagnosed positive would be different from the PET tokens he would have sent earlier in his app's ESR_REQUESTs.

2.6.3.2 Initial Registration

At the time of initial registration of the app, an Authorization Token (AT) is generated at the server end and sent to the user's phone number via SMS. This AT is used by the app to register at the backend. The phone number is not stored by the server.

The server also generates an encryption key (EK) specific to the user's app, encrypts all the entries in IDTable corresponding to the user's permanent ID (except the ID itself) with EK, sends ID and EK to the app and finally deletes the EK.

2.6.3.3   Message Structure

DESIRE does not use any message structure (like a HELLO message), instead it proposes the direct sending of EBIDs in the broadcast payload followed by the payload in the scan/response message. Even though no time value is shared, the chance of a replay attack is minimized by converting the encounter event from an asymmetrical to a symmetrical one.

2.6.3.4   Risk Scoring

In DESIRE, the Exposure Risk Score (ERS) for every app is maintained in IDTable along with the LEPM (List of Exposed PET Metadata), and the at-risk or not-at-risk status is determined based on whether this score has crossed a threshold value (decided based on guidance of epidemiologists and health authorities).

2.6.4   Highlight and Characteristics

No personal or personally identifiable information is collected: ROBERT does not collect any personal information or personally identifiable information at the time of app installation and registration. By suggesting the usage of Mixnet or proxy or intermediate trusted server (like that of a health authority) or a dedicated hardware device at the server end, it proposes to take care of masking the network identify (like IP address) of the devices at the time of data upload corresponding to the users who are diagnosed positive. In case of DESIRE, although the phone number is collected at the time of registration for ensuring that the user has the device corresponding to the phone number, it is later deleted and not stored at the server-end.

Server and app jointly own every activity: The EBIDs (Ephemeral Bluetooth IDs) that are sent, and received by the devices as part of their HELLO messages are created at the backend server for ROBERT. For DESIRE, the EBIDs are directly generated and broadcast from the device-end. The proximity details (e.g., the EBIDs) of nearby devices are stored in each device; the identification of close-contact events, their corresponding epochs and risk scoring are all performed at the server-end. Once again, the retrieval of such information (like whether a user is at-risk or not at-risk) is done by the app. Hence, we can say that the backend server and the app jointly own every activity in ROBERT and DESIRE protocols.

Cryptographic algorithms are abundantly used: Every communication, whether between two nearby devices or between a device and the server or between two federated servers uses encryption and authentication. Both symmetric as well as asymmetric keys have been used during encryption. In ROBERT all key-exchanges are interactive in nature while in DESIRE both interactive and non-interactive key exchanges have been used.

Broadcast topology mode of BLE is used: Both ROBERT and DESIRE make use of the broadcast topology mode of the BLE protocol. Since app-level encryption and authentication are used, the transparent nature of packets in broadcast topology does not pose any security or privacy threat. On the other hand, the broadcast topology possibly ensures faster exchange of messages between devices coming in proximity as compared to the connection topology mode. However, it has been proposed that the broadcast topology be used in a different way for DESIRE as compared to that for ROBERT. In case of ROBERT, the exchange of packets could be asymmetric which means if device *A* captures the BLE packets (of a ROBERT protocol based app) from device *B* in any interaction event, it is not necessary to assume that the device *B* also should captures BLE packets from A as well (even if that happens in majority of the cases). However, in DESIRE it is mandatory to have a symmetric exchange of packets between the two devices.

Configurability and extensibility: Although it has not been described in the specification in detail, it can be inferred that both ROBERT and DESIRE have several configurable elements (e.g., duration of an epoch, contagious period, tolerable time difference of a received message from current network time, risk scoring algorithm, user notification flag reset procedure etc.) that can be modified at the time of initial installation of the system or at a later point of time.

DESIRE is more decentralized than ROBERT: In DESIRE, there is no longer a dependency on the server to generate the Ephemeral Bluetooth IDs. The mobile devices generate such pseudorandom IDs independently for sending to each other and store those in such a fashion (using a non-interactive key exchange protocol) that those can be transparently matched at the server end to identify the possible close-contact events without any possibility of recovering the original pseudorandom EBIDs that got exchanged between the original devices, which came in close proximity to each other.

2.6.5   System Analysis

We divide the analysis of ROBERT and DESIRE in two parts—first we focus on the security and privacy analysis of the frameworks, and next we concentrate on the architecture analysis of the systems. We point out the possible open areas within each of these parts.

2.6.5.1 Security and Privacy Analysis

Let us first look at the system parameters, message encodings and cryptographic primitives used in ROBERT in each of the following subsections and then highlight the changes in DESIRE.

System Parameters
The system parameters are as follows:

- $T_{ptsstart}$: Start time of the proximity tracing service in the country to which the backend server belongs. It is expressed as the NTP (Network Time Protocol) *seconds* value [23]. The server also maintains an epoch number that starts with the value 0 for the first *epoch_duration_sec* duration (usually 15 min translated to number of seconds) starting from $T_{ptsstart}$. DESIRE does not mention this parameter.
- epoch_duration_sec: This is a configurable parameter that represents the duration of an epoch in seconds for the entire system.
- Delta (δ): Time tolerance for acceptability of a HELLO packet. It can typically be a few seconds. This is not applicable for DESIRE as Time is not sent as part of the message packet.
- ContStart$_A$ and ContEnd$_A$: These are derived values (in seconds) for a user A's start time (ContStart$_A$) and end time (ContEnd$_A$) of being contagious. The derivation algorithm would use a configurable parameter (CT) for the number of days (like 14 days or 21 days) as per the guidance from epidemiologists or the health authority.
- M: The number of epochs between two consecutive requests from app end to the server for getting the next set of (EBID, ECC) pairs. This is not applicable for DESIRE.
- T: The minimum number of epochs that must elapse between the consecutive ESR_REQUEST messages from the app to the server. This should be applicable for DESIRE as well. However, the specification has not commented on this.

Message encodings
The codes used in different messages are as follows:

- CC_S: Publicly known 8-bit country code values for the countries that agree to participate in the federated system around the protocol (ROBERT or DESIRE). In the HELLO messages this code is used in an encrypted form (described later) and is called the Encrypted Country Code (ECC) which is also of 8-bit length. This code is not applicable for DESIRE as it is silent about the usage of Federated system of servers.
- UN_A: A flag (called User Notified) that can have either a *true* or *false* value. When the user for app A is notified to be at-risk, this flag is set to *true*.
- LEE_A: This a list maintained for app$_A$ to contain the list of epochs in which the user corresponding to the app$_A$ got exposed to someone who later was diagnosed to be positive. In case of DESIRE the two lists that are important at server end are—the global EList (Exposure List) and the user specific LEPM$_A$ (List of Exposed PET Metadata).

- Request type: There are four types of requests and their corresponding codes. HELLO message has code 1, ESR_REQUEST has code 2, Unregister has code 3 and DeleteHistory has code 4. Among these, Unregister and DeleteHistory have not been described in the specification. For DESIRE, ESR_REQUEST is applicable, however no other message type/code has been described.

Cryptographic items

The different keys and items are as follows:

- K_S: L-bit long (where $L \geq 128$) server key (initialized during server set-up) that is used by the server to generate the EBIDs. This primitive is not applicable for DESIRE.
- K_G: L-bit long (where $L \geq 128$) federation key shared among the backend servers of the countries participating in the federated agreement. This primitive is not applicable for DESIRE.
- (sk_S, pk_S): An asymmetric key-pair (called the *registration key-pair*) where sk_S is the secret key known only to the server and pk_S is the public key distributed to all the apps. This registration key-pair is generated at the server set-up time over the elliptic curve NIST-P256 [15], where $pk_S = sk_S \cdot G$, where G signifies the base point on the prime order of the indicated elliptic curve. This key-pair is also a necessary ingredient to form a *SharedSecret* between the server and a particular instance of the app, which we describe next. This primitive is not applicable for DESIRE.
- SharedSecret: User's app (A) generates an ephemeral asymmetric key-pair $(ske_A, pke_A = ske_A \cdot G)$ and then transmits pke_A to the server. app A computes $ske_A \cdot pk_S$, while the server generates $sk_S \cdot pke_A$. Clearly, both are the same and this primitive forms the SharedSecret between the app A and the server. This primitive is not applicable for DESIRE.
- $K - Auth_A$: This is the authentication key (of length ≥ 128 bits) that is used to authenticate app A messages and both the server and the app side generates it from the SharedSecret by $K - Auth_A = \text{HMAC\_SHA256}(\text{SharedSecret, "authentication key"})$. This primitive is not applicable for DESIRE. However, an encryption key called EK is generated and shared to app A by the server.
- $K - Enc_A$: This is the encryption key (of length ≥ 128 bits) that is used to encrypt sensitive messages sent by the server to app A and both the server and the app side generates it from the SharedSecret by $K - Enc_A = \text{HMAC\_SHA256}(\text{Shared Secret}, \text{encryption key})$. This primitive is not applicable for DESIRE.
- ERS_A: Exposure Risk Score (ERS) would be maintained at server end for each registered app (A) in DESIRE. This is not mentioned in ROBERT specification.
- ID_A: This is a 40-bit unique identifier generated by the server (for both ROBERT and DESIRE based systems) using a random drawing process (without replacement) to uniquely identify app A and is not shared with app A.
- $HELLO_A$: We now dissect the encoding structure of a HELLO message emitted by the app A at an epoch i. The $HELLO_A$ message consists of an information

part (M_A of length 88 bits) and a Message Authentication Code part (MAC_A of length 40 bits). This primitive is not applicable for DESIRE.

Now we have the following process:

$$HELLO_A = [M_A | MAC_A]$$
$$MAC_A = \text{HMAC\_SHA256}(K - Auth_A, 00001111 | M_A)$$
$$M_A = [ECC_A, EBID_A, Time]$$
$$ECC_A = MSB(AES(K_G, EBID_A | 0^{64})) \oplus CC_A$$
$$EBID_A = ENC(K_S, i | ID_A), \text{ where ENC is a 64-bit block cipher}$$

Here $Time$ is less significant 16 bits of the current system time (NTP *Seconds*) and ENC can be implemented as SKINNY-64/192 [14].

Security and privacy issues

The security and privacy of the framework can be analyzed by referring to the above primitives and by considering the following adversarial models of attacks.

- **Backend impersonation:** Since the backend server would have a well-known domain name with proper certification and the communication channel between the app and the server is secured, backend impersonation attack would not be feasible by a malicious third party.
- **Server data breach:** In case of ROBERT, server data breach may have a risk of disclosing certain sensitive information like LEE list in the IDTable (although the user details like ID is a pseudonym). However, in case of DESIRE the risk is even lesser as all IDTable entries are encrypted by the EK_A keys that are known only to the corresponding apps.
- **Replay attack:** As the HELLO message contains a Time field and the entire message is protected against any tampering by using a MAC, a replay attack cannot be mounted against ROBERT. For DESIRE based systems, the symmetric exchange of PET tokens would prevent any replay attack.
- **Relay attack:** The specifications of ROBERT and DESIRE do not mention any measure against relay attacks. This could be feasible, however it may be feasible only within a limited time-span.
- **Deanonymization of users:** No personal or personally identifiable information is collected either by the app or by the server. Hence, even if the data at any end gets compromised or leaked, it would not lead to deanonymization of users. However, there could be other means (like side-channel attacks through contextual information beyond what is captured in ROBERT or DESIRE framework) through which deanonymization can still happen. One-entry attack can also lead to deanonymization. However, the extent of this attack would be limited as the system does not allow an app to send any subsequent ESR_REQUEST message once its UN flag is set to 'true' at the server end unless it is later reset through a certain approval process (not outlined in the specifications).

- **Inverse-Sybil attack:** Since the system does not verify the actual device or SIM card number to authenticate the messages between the app and the server, the inverse-Sybil attack is feasible in ROBERT but not in DESIRE (due to symmetric nature of the contact events being recorded through PET tokens).
- **Coercion threats:** For ROBERT, the data stored in a device based on the exchange of HELLO messages are not decipherable without the help of the server, hence the chance of coercion threats in these systems is limited. However, there could still be a chance of an infected person's device being misused by a malicious third party (before he/she uploads the proximity data to the server) by deliberately bringing that device in proximity to a large number of people and thereby triggering many false alarms as those users may get notified to be at-risk by the server once the data gets uploaded. The latter issue is applicable to DESIRE as well.

2.6.5.2 Possible Open Areas

We have already discussed that the protocols do not currently guard against certain attacks like relay attacks, inverse-Sybil attacks etc. as described in the previous subsection. That is, there are certain open areas that might need to be studied in a disciplined manner in future.

- The ROBERT specification does not mention the exact algorithm for generating (ID_A).
- The ROBERT specification does not mention whether the server key (K_S) is generated as a pseudo-random number.
- The ROBERT specification does not mention how the federation key (K_G) is generated and shared among the federated servers.
- The DESIRE specification does not mention how the Encryption Key (EK_A) for each app is generated by the server.
- (In ROBERT) No information shared on the choice of NIST-P256 for asymmetric registration key-pair generation on the server side, on the choice of HMAC_SHA256 for generation of $K - Auth_A$ and $K - Enc_A$ on both the server side and app side, on the choice of AES in ECC, on the choice of SKINNY-64/192 in EBID and the choice of HMAC_SHA256 in MAC generation.
- (In DESIRE) No information has been shared on the choice of Curve25519. Also, it has not been mentioned why SHA-256 has been used for the cryptographic hash function while generating the two types of PET tokens.

2.6.5.3 Architecture Analysis

Bluetooth Low Energy layer used in broadcast topology: This ensures that the communication is "easy or fast to use" [36]. Since the message size is longer than what can fit in a single broadcast packet, subsequent packets must be requested by the receiver from the broadcasting device (using Scan/Response or Fragmentation approach).

Secured communication at app level: The app uses security and authentication measures on every communication to preserve privacy and security of information.

Precaution against identification of users by the server while uploading the proximity data: The server is designed to not know who uploaded what part of the proximity data. In case of DESIRE the device end EBIDs are completely unlinkable to the server as it can only observe the PET tokens.

Simple interaction among federated servers: The federated system of servers are expected to function independently and the data exchange is kept minimal to pass information corresponding to only those users who might have traveled from one country to another, came in close contact with another user from the visited country and later at least one of them is diagnosed as positive.

2.6.5.4 Possible Open Areas

- Two message types—Unregister and DeleteHistory have not been described in ROBERT specification.
- It is not clear how DESIRE can be extended to multiple authorities.
- It is not mentioned how UN_A can be reset in the ROBERT framework once it is set (to *true*). This has been described in greater detail in the DESIRE specifications.
- (In ROBERT) If a user's app crashes and the user does a fresh registration after installing the app again, would the previous permanent ID be linkable to the present permanent ID? If not, would the previous history of LEE be lost from the user's perspective?
- (In ROBERT) Once UN is set (to *true*) for a particular user (say A), the specification mentions that her app would keep on sending HELLO messages to nearby devices. However, nothing is mentioned on whether her app would continue to receive and store HELLO messages from other devices. That would be important from A's perspective as there could be a chance of her being diagnosed as negative while some other user whose device came in close proximity to her (after A's UN flag being set as 'true') is later tested positive.
- The calibration of signal strengths for different manufacturers' devices in the broadcast topology would be critical for the success of such systems.
- The specifications talk about other metadata like signal strength or duration being used in the risk scoring algorithm, but it has not elaborated on how that would be captured.
- In Fig. 1 of the ROBERT specification [20], C is assumed to infect A as C is diagnosed positive before A gets diagnosed. However, that need not be true. A might have infected C and the symptoms shown by C might have appeared before it happened for A, which may have led C to be tested before A.
- In ROBERT's specification [20] as well as in DESIRE [12], the terms *at-risk* and *at risk of exposure* have been used interchangeably. However, *at-risk* may typically mean *at risk of being infected*, which is different from *at risk of exposure*.

- In Sect. 2.1 of ROBERT's specification [20], it is mentioned that the risk score is a binary number (*at-risk* or *not at risk*). However, that call should only be taken at the medical personnel level. For example, the same duration and proximity of exposure of a person with another infected individual may be considered to have different levels of risk based on the age of the user. For a young asymptomatic individual, a health advisor may not suggest immediate testing to be done—however, if the person is aged (although asymptomatic so far), the guidance could be different. So only communicating a binary value would be too limiting for a medical professional to take a call on what needs to be done. This issue may arise in case of DESIRE protocol as well.
- It appears that once an application is labeled *at risk*—it remains in that state forever. However, in reality that would not be the case. If A and C came in close contact 14 days back and C is tested positive today, A can be falsely considered at-risk the present time (day) and not anymore from tomorrow. So if C's application notifies the server of the fact that C is tested positive and A's application is marked at-risk today, if A's application happens to not be running at the present day and it wakes up tomorrow and sends an exposure status request to the server tomorrow—the server should not declare A to be at-risk. How is this checked in the system? There can also be cumulative effects of exposure of an individual repeatedly over a number of days—it may not be fair to record that as one instance of *at-risk*.

2.7 Conclusion

In this chapter we have discussed some of the contact tracing protocols in details, mostly from the aspects how a centralized server participates in such designs. That is, we have considered the centralized systems in this chapter. The basic framework and protocol details are discussed. We describe the BlueTrace, OpenTrace and TraceTogether protocols from different aspects. Then we consider the COVIDSafe proposal. Finally we note that the boundary between the centralized and decentralized protocols might not be very stringent in certain cases. That is why we have discussed ROBERT and DESIRE in great details that show how the designs move towards decentralized domain via the hybrid route. Based on this understanding, in the next section, we will discuss the decentralized protocols in details.

References

1. A high level overview of PEPP-PT_NTK. https://nadim.computer/res/pdf/PEPP-PT_NTK_High_Level_Overview.pdf.
2. Aarogya Setu App. https://www.mygov.in/aarogya-setu-app/.
3. Aarogya Setu App Forum. https://www.mygov.in/task/aarogya-setu-app-covid-19-tracker-launched-alert-you-and-keep-you-safe-download-now/. Aarogya Setu App.
4. Aarogya setu wikipedia page. https://en.wikipedia.org/wiki/Aarogya_Setu.

5. Angius, E., & Witte, R. (2012). OpenTrace: An open source Workbench for automatic software traceability link recovery. In *19th Working Conference on Reverse Engineering, Kingston, ON, 2012*, pp. 507–508. https://doi.org/10.1109/WCRE.2012.63.https://github.com/opentrace-community.

6. AU-COVIDSafe/mobile-android Github repository. https://github.com/AU-COVIDSafe/mobile-android.

7. AU-COVIDSafe/mobile-ios Github repository. https://github.com/AU-COVIDSafe/mobile-ios.

8. Bay, J., Kek, J., Tan, A., Hau, C. S., Yongquan, L., Tan, J., & Quy, T. A. BlueTrace: A privacy-preserving protocol for community-driven contact tracing across borders. https://bluetrace.io/static/bluetrace_whitepaper-938063656596c104632def383eb33b3c.pdf.

9. Beierle, C., Jean, J., Kölbl, S., Leander, G., Moradi, A., Peyrin, T., Sasaki, Y., Sasdrich, P., & Sim, S. M. (2016). The SKINNY family of block ciphers and its low-latency variant MANTIS. Cryptology ePrint Archive: Report 2016/660. https://eprint.iacr.org/2016/660.pdf.

10. BlueTrace protocol: Privacy-preserving cross-border contact tracing. https://bluetrace.io/.

11. Bluetooth Core Specification Version 5.1 Feature Overview. https://www.bluetooth.com/bluetooth-resources/bluetooth-core-specification-v5-1-feature-overview/.

12. Castelluccia, C., Bielova, N., Boutet, A., Cunche, M., Lauradoux, C., Le Métayer, D., & Roca, V. DESIRE: A third way for a European exposure notification system leveraging the best of centralized and decentralized systems. https://hal.inria.fr/hal-02570382/document.

13. COVIDSafe App Website by Australian Government Department of Health. https://www.health.gov.au/resources/apps-and-tools/covidsafe-app.

14. COVIDSafe application privacy impact assessment on the COVIDSafe website by Australian Government Department of Health. https://www.health.gov.au/resources/publications/covidsafe-application-privacy-impact-assessment.

15. Digital Signature Standard (DSS). FIPS PUB 186-4. *Federal Information Processing Standards Publication. Information Technology Laboratory, National Institute of Standards and Technology*. https://nvlpubs.nist.gov/nistpubs/FIPS/NIST.FIPS.186-4.pdf.

16. Firebase wikipedia page. https://en.wikipedia.org/wiki/Firebase.

17. GovTech Singapore Website. 6 things about OpenTrace, the open-source code published by the TraceTogether team. https://www.tech.gov.sg/media/technews/six-things-about-opentrace.

18. Gvili, Y. (2020). Security analysis of the COVID-19 contact tracing specifications by Apple Inc. and Google Inc. *Cryptology ePrint Archive*, Report 2020/428, 2020. https://eprint.iacr.org/2020/428.

19. Inria, France and Fraunhofer AISEC, Germany. ROBERT: ROBust and privacy-presERving proximity Tracing – Summary. https://github.com/ROBERT-proximity-tracing/documents/blob/master/ROBERT-summary-EN.pdf.

20. Inria, France and Fraunhofer AISEC, Germany. ROBERT: ROBust and privacy-presERving proximity Tracing – Specification. https://github.com/ROBERT-proximity-tracing/documents/blob/master/ROBERT-specification-EN-v1_1.pdf.

21. Inria, France and Fraunhofer AISEC, Germany. ROBERT: ROBust and privacy-presERving proximity Tracing – Documents. https://github.com/ROBERT-proximity-tracing/documents.

22. NIST Special Publication 800-38D. (2007). Recommendation for block cipher modes of operation: Galois/Counter Mode (GCM) and GMAC. *National Institute of Standards and Technology*, November, 2007.

23. Network Time Protocol Wikipedia Page. https://en.wikipedia.org/wiki/Network_Time_Protocol.

24. Next phase of NHS coronavirus (COVID-19) app announced. https://www.gov.uk/government/news/next-phase-of-nhs-coronavirus-covid-19-app-announced.

25. NHS_COVID-19 App website by the government of UK. https://www.nhsx.nhs.uk/covid-19-response/nhs-covid-19-app/.

26. nhsx/COVID-19-app-Android-BETA Github repository. https://github.com/nhsx/COVID-19-app-Android-BETA.

27. nhsx/COVID-19-app-iOS-BETA Github repository. https://github.com/nhsx/COVID-19-app-iOS-BETA.
28. Pan-European privacy-preserving proximity tracing. https://www.pepp-pt.org/.
29. Pietrzak, K. Delayed authentication replay and relay attacks on DP-3T. *Cryptology ePrint Archive*, Report 2020/418. https://eprint.iacr.org/2020/418.
30. Privacy policy for COVIDSafe app language translations on the COVIDSafe website by Australian Government Department of Health. https://www.health.gov.au/resources/translated/privacy-policy-for-covidsafe-app-other-languages.
31. Concerns on the NHS_COVID-19 wikipedia page. https://en.wikipedia.org/wiki/NHS_COVID-19#Concerns.
32. Independent analysis on the COVIDSafe wikipedia page. https://en.wikipedia.org/wiki/COVIDSafe#Independent_analysis.
33. OpenTrace on the BlueTrace wikipedia page. https://en.wikipedia.org/wiki/BlueTrace#OpenTrace.
34. The crypto group at IST Austria. Inverse-Sybil attacks in automated contact tracing. https://eprint.iacr.org/2020/670.
35. The COVIDSafe application privacy impact assessment agency response. COVIDSafe document by Australian Government Department of Health. https://www.health.gov.au/sites/default/files/documents/2020/04/covidsafe-application-privacy-impact-assessment-agency-response.pdf.
36. Townsend, K., Cufí, C., Akiba, & Davidson, R. Getting started with bluetooth low energy. https://www.oreilly.com/library/view/getting-started-with/9781491900550/ch01.html.
37. TraceTogether wikipedia page. https://en.wikipedia.org/wiki/TraceTogether.
38. Valk, R. Contact tracing apps - can we trust the tech? https://platform.deloitte.com.au/articles/contact-tracing-apps-can-we-trust-the-tech.
39. Vaudenay, S. Centralized or decentralized? The contact tracing dilemma. https://eprint.iacr.org/2020/531.
40. Vaudenay, S. Analysis of DP-3T between Scylla and Charybdis. https://eprint.iacr.org/2020/399.pdf.
41. Website of the Federal Register of Legislation, Australian Government. Biosecurity (Human biosecurity emergency) (Human coronavirus with pandemic potential) (Emergency requirements–Public health contact information) Determination 2020. https://www.legislation.gov.au/Details/F2020L00480.
42. Why the NHS Covid-19 contact tracing app failed. https://www.wired.co.uk/article/nhs-tracing-app-scrapped-apple-google-uk.
43. Wikipedia page on NHS_COVID-19. https://en.wikipedia.org/wiki/NHS_COVID-19.
44. Wikipedia page on COVID-19 Apps. https://en.wikipedia.org/wiki/COVID-19_apps.

Chapter 3
Decentralized Contact Tracing Protocols

Abstract Digital Contact Tracing (DCT) protocols and systems usually rely upon close-range communication between handheld devices (like smartphones or tablets), primarily using the Bluetooth Low Energy (BLE) interface and a client-server mode of communication between the apps installed on the devices and the backend server(s). Depending upon the role played by the backend server(s), DCT protocols, and systems are usually classified under centralized or decentralized categories. In this chapter, we focus on decentralized DCT protocols, namely, Apple-Google Exposure Notification Framework (ENF), DP3T, East Coast PACT, West Coast PACT, and TCN. Towards the end, we describe Epione, which though categorized under decentralized systems according to the classification provided in Chap. 2, contains many features akin to that of centralized systems.

3.1 Introduction

The proximity graph of a contact tracing system is one in which users are considered as vertices and any two vertices are connected by an edge if the apps of corresponding users detect the presence of each other's device in their vicinity. This graph could be directed or undirected according to whether the detection occurs in pairs of users interacting with each other (by exchanging proximity identifiers) or independently (by a broadcast of identifiers, which may be detected by other users even when the broadcasting app may not detect the receiving users) respectively. Centralized systems for contact tracing allow the central server to determine the neighborhoods of infected users; it may not always be possible or feasible to trust it with such information. This may be due to various reasons, some of which include security concerns like direct attacks on the server for access to or manipulation of bulk information from malicious entities, hardware and software capacity concerns like the possibility of overload on the server and related issues like generation of errors in the system,

© The Author(s), under exclusive license to Springer Nature Singapore Pte Ltd. 2020   71
P. Chakraborty et al., *Contact Tracing in Post-Covid World*,
Indian Statistical Institute Series,
https://doi.org/10.1007/978-981-15-9727-5_3

social and legal matters such as privacy laws in a country or lack of trust of users towards the authority that manages the server, etc. Most of these reasons, especially the last one, may discourage a large proportion of the population from participating in the app-based contact tracing process, which may adversely affect the effectiveness of such measures in controlling the spread of the disease. Thus, in addition to the problem of contact tracing with security against non-authoritative adversaries, these concerns give rise to the problem of carrying out these tasks in a manner that is also secure from entities of the central administration like the backend server and the health authorities.

The dependence on the trustworthiness of the health authority cannot be completely eliminated as the system depends on it for diagnosis and medical advice; the security measures that can be taken from a cryptographic standpoint are quite simply the implementation of precautions such as encryption of user data, authentication, and verification of data through suitable algorithms, use of blockchains, hash chains, etc., (some of these approaches also provide added layers of security against attacks from users and other entities). However, the system must undergo drastic changes to ensure security against the central server. This fundamentally requires a definition of the amount and nature of data to which the server has access, in terms of its capability to compute additional information about users (e.g., infection or diagnosis status, neighborhoods, primary or secondary contacts, location, time markers, etc.) from this data.

3.1.1 Characteristics of Decentralized Systems

The common characteristics of almost all decentralized systems are as follows.

- Any centralized agency like the Administrative Authority or the Epidemiological Authority have limited information about the users (that can be used to personally identify the individual), contact events, or identifiers being broadcast/received between the apps or devices. However, the Health Authority would have access to infected users' identities in the majority of the protocols.
- Most of the backend servers (e.g., the server that stores the list of proximity identifiers of infected users or the seeds from which these identifiers can be derived) are considered to be semi-trusted entities. The Health Authority server is considered to be a trusted one.
- If a user tests positive, then he/she would be expected to upload the proximity identifiers (that the user-app shared with the neighboring devices and/or received from such devices over the last 14 days or so) to the backend/bulletin-board server(s).
- The risk computation is mostly done at the user-app end.
- In case the server data is compromised, the extent of damage would be limited as no personal or personally identifiable user data are usually stored at the server end. In a distributed bulletin-board implementation of the server with sophisticated cryptographic algorithms, the list of random seeds/identifiers corresponding to the

infected users or the contact events can remain safe even if the data falls in the hands of malicious entities.

- Epidemiological requirements are not addressed in most of the decentralized protocols. In fact, DP3T specification explicitly puts this under out-of-scope.
- Intuitively it appears that the interoperability among the decentralized systems may be easy to achieve. However, none of the specifications elaborates a possible mechanism.
- Since most of the critical operations including evaluation of the at-risk or not at-risk status of users is carried out at device end, it may become complex to roll-out system-level changes, bug-fixes, and enhancements (e.g., modification of the risk-scoring algorithm) in decentralized systems as compared to centralized systems.

The common cryptographic primitives of such systems would be similar to those of centralized systems.

3.2 A General Framework of Decentralized Protocol

In the previous chapter, we have described centralized contact tracing protocols. Now we describe how a decentralized contact tracing protocol works. If A and B interact through a decentralized app, their time-of-contact data get stored locally in their apps through a direct broadcast, without the involvement of the server. For this reason, we call those protocols decentralized. If one of them (say A) has tested positive for SARS-CoV-2, a part of all interaction of A with other users would be reported to the server through a proper authentication channel. Any user, say B, can verify contact with A by matching the reported interaction with his own stored interaction. Thus, the role of the central server in any decentralized protocol is to facilitate through its database/bulletin board, the communication between an infected user with all other users.

In Chap. 1, we have described different phases of a DCTS. Here, we focus on the features that are specific to decentralized systems.

1. **Registration and Initialization Phase:** At the time of registration and initialization, the user-app would generate the first set of seeds/keys from which the proximity identifiers (as well as the subsequent daily or hourly seeds) would be formed. There would be no involvement of the backend server(s) in this activity.
2. **Contact-Broadcast Phase:** There is no difference in this phase between the centralized and decentralized systems/protocols.
3. **Reporting Phase:** If at any point of time, A tests positive, A's app sends some information to the central authority. This authority uses a server to broadcast this information, which may be encrypted by a public key or maintained in a blockchain for added security. Alternatively, symmetric key generation and encryption using such keys can also be implemented.

4. **Risk-level (or Risk-score) Computation Phase:** Different apps that receive
   this information (automatically at regular intervals, or manually through user-
   generated requests) use a verification algorithm to check whether they had indeed
   come into contact with A using the broadcast information obtained from the
   server and the key(s) shared directly with A.

Below we describe the possible attack scenarios that could be mounted by various
types of malicious users (or user groups), which every decentralized DCTS must be
prepared to handle in a graceful manner.

3.2.1 Attack Scenarios

In the case of decentralized digital contact tracing systems, servers and communication channels can be considered to be less vulnerable as compared to the centralized
systems, due to minimal roles played by the non-user entities. Hence, such systems
can be envisaged to have stronger cryptographic safeguards. However, errors in communication, heavy traffic, overloading, etc. (because of genuine reasons or malicious
adversaries), cannot be completely ruled out. Thus, false negatives, linkage attacks
and DoS attacks may still occur as a consequence of these factors.

The designated health agencies who have the testing authority are also expected
to guide patients through diagnosis, evaluation of exposure risks, etc. The possible
misuse of these functions by a corrupt health authority, even though may happen in
reality, cannot be cryptographically controlled. Hence, for the purpose of security
analysis, we would consider the Health Authority as a trusted entity. In the following
subsections, we would consider the attack scenarios mainly from the context of
DP3T, Apple-Google Framework, East Coast PACT, West Coast PACT, and TCN.

3.2.1.1 Integrity Attacks Through False Positives

Adversaries may execute replay attacks by either broadcasting identifiers of infected
individuals as soon as they are uploaded to the server or by creating a pool of (false)
identifiers and broadcasting them to unknowing users. The first attack can be averted
by simply securing the communication channels to the server. The second attack
is only successful if the pool of false identifiers contains some matches with the
identifiers uploaded by infected users; it can be easily prevented by timestamping all
identifiers. However, care must be taken to keep the timestamps as coarse as possible
as the inclusion of exact times could lead to loss of privacy. Another way to avoid
replay attacks is to replace the broadcasting of identifiers by an interactive protocol
between two users coming into contact with each other for authentication.

Relay attacks are stronger than replay attacks as they can circumvent timestamping
and other measures that could deal with replay attacks. Implementation of distance-
bounding protocols, inclusion of a coarse location-stamp through GPS, etc., can be

used to mitigate relay attacks. Distance-bounding is more difficult to implement and could lower the privacy of users. Implementing an interactive protocol between two users along with a binding commitment scheme (as proposed for DP3T in [38]) is another solution, albeit costly.

An inverse-Sybil attack can be executed on such protocols, possibly on a large scale, by collecting the identifiers broadcasted by infected users (before or after uploading to the server), and further broadcasting them to other users. A malicious entity could pay users for such information if the identifiers provided by them are indeed uploaded to the server. Use of timestamping and distance-bounding protocols together could be a means to evade the inverse-Sybil attack, but this is certainly costly. Encrypting the data on the server could inconvenience an adversary wanting to check the uploads on the server, but would not prevent this attack. Involvement of the health authority for authentication and upload of identifiers of positively tested users could reduce the extensiveness of this attack.

False reports of infection could be sent to the server by malicious users, but this can be easily mitigated in various ways such as running the user-app on a Trusted Platform Module (TPM), authenticating the identifiers (or keys or seeds) uploaded by the users through the health authority or strictly restricting the uploads to the health authority (on consent from the user) and accepting identifier sets only in acceptable sizes according to the length of the infection period.

3.2.1.2   Integrity Attacks Through False Negatives

As users have the choice of not uploading their keys even on positive testing, some malicious users could accomplish a basic false negative attack by refusing to upload (some, all or correct values of) their identifiers to the server even on infection. An honest infected user may be forced to behave like this under coercion. Other reasons for false negatives could be fluctuations in Bluetooth signal strengths, incorrect evaluation, DoS attack, etc.

3.2.1.3   Privacy Attacks

Privacy of users may be compromised if the decentralized systems are subjected to a linkage attack, deanonymization attack, single-entry attack, address carryover attack, shared carryover attack, etc. Sending alerts to exposed users after an acceptable amount of time delay could be a possible way to work around some of these attacks. Other methods such as randomly permuting the identifiers received could also be employed. As all protocols discussed here involve some kind of proximity identifiers (pseudonymous and pseudorandom numbers), an important point of consideration is the frequency at which these identifiers must be changed. Tracking of BLE MAC addresses could lead to deanonymization or linkage attacks if performed on a system with a lower frequency of change.

3.3   DP-PPT/DP3T

Decentralized Privacy-Preserving Proximity Tracing (DP3T/DP-3T) is a protocol and framework proposed by a group of researchers, technologists, engineers, epidemiologists, and legal experts from a number of institutions and organizations. The list of affiliations of the team and the entire set of documents are included in the Github repository [14]. The team has also released the reference implementations of the app and the server code in the open-source domain [15, 16]. The "Who we are" page [14] clarifies that DP3T is a "free-standing effort." Although some of its members are part of the umbrella organization called Pan-European Privacy-Preserving Proximity Testing (PEPP-PT) project, it would be incorrect, as per the DP3T team, to use the term PEPP-PT for any particular protocol (e.g., DP3T), since there is a drastic difference in the approach of DP3T with some of the other centralized protocols endorsed by PEPP-PT.

For the purpose of this section, we primarily refer to the most recent white paper [11] published by the group, dated 25 May 2020.

3.3.1   Framework and Design Principles

The DP3T repository includes a set of documents that describe protocol specifications, recommendations, analyses, and comparative study (with respect to other protocol specifications like BlueTrace, PEPP-PT NTK, ROBERT, DESIRE, etc.). The current version of the white paper [11] describes three variations of a decentralized protocol, called—(1) the low-cost design, (2) the unlinkable design, and (3) the hybrid design. Apart from this main document, the repository contains an Interoperability Specification [17], an analysis of Privacy and Security Attacks [18], the Upload Authorization Analysis and Guidelines [19], the Exposure Score Calculation [20], etc.

In scope and out-of-scope areas: The specification [11] highlights that the purpose of the protocol and the framework is to complement (and not replace) the manual contact tracing process through a smartphone-based digital proximity tracing system by providing "a mechanism that alerts users who have been in close physical proximity to a confirmed COVID-19 positive case for a prolonged duration that they may have been exposed to the virus." The aims of the DP3T project are documented in [12].

Interestingly, it also points out the out-of-scope areas (called non-goals), like (a) tracking of users who have been diagnosed positive (b) identify the hotspot areas or the trajectories of infected cases, and (c) sharing any data for epidemiological research purposes. The last point (about not sharing any data for research) might have some disagreement with certain statements in the Simplified Overview document [13], like "epidemiologists obtain an anonymized proximity graph with minimal information."

The system requirements of DP3T framework have been grouped under the following categories.

- **Proximity tracing requirements:** (a) Completeness (implying that all close proximity events are captured), (b) Precision (which means reported events correspond to the close proximity events), (c) Authenticity (e.g., users cannot fake exposure events), (d) Confidentiality (e.g., contact history would not get compromised or leaked), and (e) Notification (i.e., individuals can be informed about exposure risk through the system).
- **Digital privacy rights and data protection requirements:** For example, adherence to European General Data Protection Regulations [31], etc.
- **Scalability and interoperability requirements:** This is to ensure that the system can be used for the pandemic for a long period of time (if needed) at a global scale.
- **Technical feasibility requirements:** The system should not rely on new technological breakthroughs and should be deployable over a wide variety of hardware types (as mobile devices).

In spite of declaring these system requirements in an explicit fashion, the document does not validate, analyze, or study these properties on the proposed protocol for any of the three variations of the design. Surprisingly, there is no mention of the words like "Completeness" or "Precision" in the entire white paper apart from the "System requirements" section.

3.3.2 Protocol Details

We now describe the protocol details for the three design variations as proposed in the current version [11] of the specification. In all the designs, the proximity identifier is referred to as the ephemeral ID (EphID).

Low-cost design: A random 32-byte seed (SK_t) is generated on the first day (t) as per UTC convention of days and on every day thereafter a new secret seed is generated as $SK_{t+1} = H(SK_t)$, where H is a cryptographic hash function. A day is divided in L-minute-long fixed durations called the epochs. For the entire day, a list of n EphIDs are generated, where n equals $(\frac{24 \cdot 60}{L})$ in the following manner:

$$\text{EphID}_1 || \ldots || \text{EphID}_n = \text{PRG}(\text{PRF}(SK_t, \text{"broadcast key"})),$$

where PRF is a pseudorandom function like HMAC-SHA256 and PRG is a pseudorandom generator (e.g., AES in counter mode). The user-app randomly picks one of the n EphIDs for each epoch and broadcasts the same in that duration. When an app receives one such EphID inside a broadcast BLE packet, it stores the same in local app-storage with the signal attenuation indicator and the day (like "July 10").

This results in a storage requirement of typically 6.1 MB, for a period of 14 days. In addition, the app also stores the SK_t values for a period of 14 days (which is a configurable parameter that is set as per recommendations from the epidemiologists). When a user is diagnosed positive, he may choose to upload (after receiving relevant authorization/validation from the Health Authority), the (SK_t, t) pair corresponding to the starting day from when he could have been contagious. After uploading is done, the infected user's app chooses a new random key as the starting secret key to generate the EphIDs from that day onwards. Each user-app on a regular interval downloads the list of such pairs corresponding to the infected users from the backend and derives the subsequent EphIDs to check for any match in the local database and determine the extent of exposure by referring to the associated metadata like signal attenuation and date.

Unlinkable design: In this approach, the smartphone draws a random 32-byte seed (seed$_i$) for the epoch i and sets EphID$_i$ = LEFTMOST128(H(seed$_i$)), where LEFTMOST128 takes the leftmost 128 bits from the output of the cryptographic hash function H. The user-app stores all the generated seeds in the past 14 days or so. When an app receives a broadcast BLE beacon, it stores a hashed version of the received EphID in the forms of H(EphID $\parallel i$), where H is the cryptographic hash function and i is the epoch number in which the beacon was received. Like the low-cost design, the app also stores the signal attenuation and the day (like "July 10"). This results in a storage requirement of typically 6.9 MB, for a period of 14 days. In this design, the app allows an infected user to redact some of the entries to be uploaded to the backend server by choosing a subset (I) of epochs from the entire period for which he could be contagious. The list of (seed$_i$, i) pairs for all i-values that belong to the set I are then uploaded to the server which periodically (every 2 h) runs through such sets and creates a new 'Cuckoo' filter (F) that includes H(LEFTMOST128(H(seed$_i$)) $\parallel i$) entry for every (seed$_i$, i) pair. Every user-app downloads the list of new Cuckoo filters and checks if there is any match against the received EphID entries stored in its local database. This ensures that the actual EphIDs of the infected users do not get revealed to any other user in the system. The parameters of the Cuckoo filter is designed in such a way that there is a very low probability of False Positives (like one in a million users who could be using the system for over 5 years). The exposure detection algorithm in this design is identical to that of the low-cost design.

Hybrid design: As the name suggests, this is a hybrid of the low-cost and the unlinkable designs. In this design, a new secret seed is generated afresh in a time-window (w) which could typically be 2–4 h long and may range from 10 min to 1 day. The relationship of the epoch duration (L) with w and n (the number of EphIDs in a time window w) is given by $n = \frac{w}{L}$. The 16-byte long EphIDs are generated as follows:

$$\text{EphID}_{w,1} \parallel \ldots \parallel \text{EphID}_{w,n} = \text{PRG}(\text{PRF}(\text{seed}_w, \text{"DP3T} - \text{HYBRID"})),$$

where PRF is a pseudorandom function like HMAC-SHA256 and PRG is a pseudo-random generator like AES in counter mode. When an app receives one such EphID inside a broadcast BLE packet, it stores the same in local app-storage with the signal attenuation indicator and the day (like "July 10")—this is similar to the approach used in the low-cost design. This results in a storage requirement of typically 4.8 MB, for a period of 14 days. When a user is diagnosed positive, he would have the option to redact certain entries before uploading the seeds to the server after necessary authorization from the Health Authority. The exposure detection step by matching the downloaded seeds from the server and the exposure detection algorithm are identical to that of the low-cost design. The specification has mentioned that if the value of w is equal to 1 day (in minutes), the design would appear similar to that of the Apple-Google Exposure Notification Framework.

3.3.3 Highlights and Characteristics

Some of the highlights and characteristics of the DP3T framework are as follows.

- It has assimilated a diverse set of elements and parameters in the three design variations. Hence, the framework may work out very differently for the three approaches when it comes to implementation trade-offs or user experience.
- The framework is focused on keeping the footprints of data stores (at device and server end) and device to server communications small so that the bandwidth usage and latency can be minimized. It has also published details of estimated data sizes and the requirements of daily data download size for each of its three design variations in multiple European countries. To the best of our knowledge, no other protocol or framework has gone to this extent of analysis in terms of bandwidth usage and data requirements. The specification has analyzed the security and privacy considerations for the three design variations under different threat models in an extensive fashion. It has also published separate documents that study the security and privacy for decentralized systems in a generic way as well as presented specific security and privacy analyses for some of the other protocols, including PEPP-PT, ROBERT, DESIRE, etc. The document repository also includes a note that addresses the possible alternate ways and mechanisms on how the Health Authority may validate the infected user's status.
- The specification also touches upon the multi-country or multi-state interoperability considerations for apps based on the DP3T protocol and the overview of a mechanism for an integrated exposure computation based on per-day exposure score.
- The "Readme" file [14] refers to the Apple-Google Exposure Notification Framework and has mentioned that "DP-3T appreciates the endorsement of these two companies for our solution and has been working with both of them to implement our app on their platforms"—it would be worthwhile to watch this space to see further developments that may come out through such a collaboration.

3.3.4   System Analysis

Since the basic system analysis has already been discussed in the previous subsections, let us go directly to the security and architecture analyses of the protocol.

3.3.4.1   Security Analysis

The following discussion is primarily inspired by the extensive analysis of DP3T done by Vaudenay in his well-referred paper [38]. However, the DP3T specification has also evolved over time and its proposed design approaches have been refined based on many of the comments and suggestions posted in the Github forum. The current version of the white paper also highlights most of these attack scenarios.

- **Backend impersonation:** The possibility of backend impersonation may not be ruled out and it would depend on the level of security and certification followed for the server that is expected to publish the seeds or Cuckoo filters corresponding to the infected users. Irrespective of which of the three designs are followed in the implementation, a malicious backend server can cause harm by sharing incorrect seeds/filters with the apps, which would generate a large-scale False Negatives.
- **Server data breach:** The backend server does not store any user-specific personal or personally identifiable information. Hence, even if there is a data breach at the server end, there would be no serious risk of losing sensitive data. However, there could be a considerable risk of deanonymization of infected users who have uploaded their seeds to the server.
- **Replay attack:** In the low-cost design, there is a high chance of replay attack within a duration of a day. In the other two designs, this could be feasible within the duration of an epoch (L minutes).
- **Relay attack:** DP3T is not resistant to relay attacks (although engineering such an attack is always cumbersome for an adversary) for all the three design variations.
- **Deanonymization of users:** Since the seeds/filters corresponding to the infected users are directly downloaded by every user-app, deanonymization can be implemented by malicious users or user groups in all the three design variations. Such users may arrange to passively listen to EphIDs of users (along with additional information like captured images of people who would have come near the beacon capturing devices), especially in places where the density of infected users is expected to be high (like in hospitals) and matching those against the EphIDs generated from the seeds (or running those through the Cuckoo filters). Single-entry attacks can also lead to deanonymization.
- **Inverse-Sybil attack:** DP3T is not resistant to such attacks as there is no permanent identifier of the user that is attached to a particular device identifier (SIM number or IMEI number) for any of the three design variations.
- **Coercion threats:** DP3T is also susceptible to such attacks irrespective of the design variation used. An infected person's device can be misused by a malicious third party (before he/she uploads the proximity data to the server) by deliberately

bringing that device in proximity to a large number of people, which would trigger many false alarms in the ecosystem.

- **Miscellaneous:** DP3T is susceptible to Denial of Service (DoS) attack and many other generic mobile device's OS or API layer attacks. In the white paper, it is mentioned as a footnote that MAC address change is assumed to be synchronized with the EphID change in BLE messages. If that does not happen properly, the protocol can be susceptible to address carryover attacks. There is no mention of message authentication at the BLE protocol layer. Hence, it is not clear how DP3T may resist message tampering attempts at the lowermost level.

3.3.4.2 Architecture Analysis

We now describe some of the possible open areas in the DP3T architecture.

- **Fault tolerance:** The specification has not talked about the login-id/user-id generation process. If a user's app crashes and the user registers afresh to the system after installing the app again, would the previous user-id be linkable to the new user-id? If not, would the previous history of exposure be lost forever?
- **Background/foreground mode:** It is not specified if the app needs to run in foreground or background mode in different platforms so that it may function effectively.
- **Interoperability:** The interoperability specification talks about multi-country implementation of systems/frameworks based on the DP3T protocol; however, there is no mention of how multiple decentralized protocols or multiple centralized as well as decentralized systems may work together.

3.4 Apple-Google Exposure Notification Framework

Google and Apple have jointly developed a digital contact tracing protocol and a system of APIs, together called the Exposure Notification Framework (ENF) [22] that can support both Android and iOS devices. It is a decentralized protocol and has a lot of similarities with the DP3T [11] and TCN [10] specifications. The most significant difference of this framework with any other system is a tight integration of the APIs at the OS level that not only makes the APIs efficient but also allows any app that uses these APIs function effectively in the background mode, even when the device is locked. No other automated contact tracing protocol or system currently has this capability.

3.4.1 Framework

In case of earlier releases, users required an app to access the Exposure Notification APIs. These apps need to be approved by Google and Apple and the approval is given only to the apps that belong to public health authorities. In the current release of ENF, Google, and Apple have developed Exposure Notification Express that integrates the core functionality in the form of a custimizable app (for Android) or at the OS layer (for iOS), so that users may be able to benefit from the features even without installing any contact racing app.

The complete list of criteria [33] that an app must meet to qualify for Google and Apple's approval is as follows.

- The app must belong to a Government Health Agency that acts as the Health Authority in a given jurisdiction and must be deemed to be part of the authority's response to the COVID-19 situation
- The app must explicitly seek user's consent for accessing the APIs and for running in the background
- It must require user's explicit consent before sharing any app-data or device-data with the backend server(s) when a user is diagnosed as positive (called the "affected user" in ENF)
- The app should gather minimal personal or personally identifiable data and any data collected should only be used for COVID-19 purpose and not for any other purpose (like an advertisement)
- Such an app must not access any geo-location information and should not seek consent from the user to have location access. In case, any existing DCT app has access to the geo-location data, it would not be able to utilize Exposure Notification APIs.
- One country can have only one such officially approved app unless that country has a federated state-based structure where each state is entitled to follow a separate approach (like the states of the USA) in which case the approval would be separately given for each state's designated app.

ENF uses BLE in the broadcast (non-connectable) topology mode. The MAC addresses stored in the BLE broadcast packets are changed synchronously with the changing proximity identifiers.

3.4.2   Design Principle

Some of the design principles that have been highlighted by Google and Apple in their documentations [2], are as follows.

- A core design principle is to maintain the user's security and privacy. This is achieved at multiple layers. In the API layers, this is ensured through the cryptologic primitives and algorithms. The decentralized architecture takes care of the fact that the backend server has a limited knowledge about user status and contact events. The computation of exposure risk happens entirely at the device end. The qualifying criteria for the apps (as described in the previous subsection) provides users a better control over the security and privacy of their own data. A user's choice plays a key role in how the app functions in his/her device.

- The specification is not dependent on any personal or personally identifiable data to be entered by the user (like phone number)
- Location metadata is not allowed to be tracked or stored in any form
- Google and Apple may also disable the service in any country or region once it is no longer required
- Both the companies are committed to not monetize the data exchanged as part of this framework
- Each public health authority may customize the parameters to define the way the app (based on ENF) may be used in that jurisdiction. This includes the way the app would determine the exposure risk (e.g., the minimum duration for which two devices must be near to each other to be recognized as an exposure event can vary between 5 and 30 min), the number of days beyond which the device data would automatically get deleted, the content of the notification message when an individual is identified by the app as a *potentially exposed user*, the look and feel of the app, etc.

3.4.3 Protocol Details

We describe the protocol in three parts as per the documented [1] specifications—(1) the Bluetooth Specification, (2) the Cryptography Specification, and (3) the Framework API.

3.4.3.1 Bluetooth Specification

The proximity identifiers are referred to as Rolling Proximity Identifiers (RPI) in this protocol. These identifiers are derived every day from a Temporary Exposure Key (TEK) and RPIs are changed every 15 min. TEKs are changed once every 24 h. The version of the protocol and the device's transmit power are stored as the Associated Encrypted Metadata (AEM). AEM is also changed every 15 min along with the RPI. The exposure notification service is registered with the Bluetooth Special Interest Group (Bluetooth SIG) as a service 0xFD6F (Service UUID). The advertising payload contains 22-byte Service Data that includes 2 bytes of Service UUID, 16 bytes of RPI, and 4 bytes of AEM. The transmitted power level is encoded as part of the AEM and has a length of 1 byte.

We have already mentioned earlier that the BLE needs to operate in Broadcast Topology mode in ENF. The recommended broadcasting interval as per specification is 200–270 milliseconds, however, it can be changed. When a device acts as the observer, it receives the RPIs from nearby devices and stores the same along with the time-stamps and signal strength values (RSSI values). The recommended scanning strategy is expected to be opportunistic where it should leverage the existing wake-up and scan intervals.

Whenever the app hands over the downloaded set of diagnostic keys (corresponding to the users who have been tested positive) to the Bluetooth layer, it picks up each of the stored RPIs and passes on that to the crypto layer along with each individual diagnosis key to determine if there has been any match or not. In the process of interaction to determine the exposure risk, the Bluetooth protocol layer acts as the intermediary between the app and the crypto API-layer.

3.4.3.2 Cryptologic Specifications

Time is discretized in 10-min intervals starting from the Unix Epoch Time and then every time interval is converted to a number (i) representing the count of intervals from that starting time. The TEK is generated as $TEK_i = CRNG(16)$, where CRNG stands for a cryptographic random number generator and 16 stands for the number of bytes in the desired random number. TEK is regenerated after 144 time intervals (i.e., 24 h).

The Rolling Proximity Identifier Key (RPIK) is derived from TEK using the computation $RPIK_i = HKDF(TEK_i, NULL, UTF8(\text{"EN-RPIK"}), 16)$, where HKDF is a SHA-256 hash function as per RFC 5869. The Rolling Proximity Identifier (RPI) at a Unix Epoch Time j is derived from RPIK as per $RPI_{i,j} = AES128(RPIK_i, PaddedData_j)$, where $PaddedData_j$ is dependent upon the time interval value corresponding to j.

Similarly, Associated Encrypted Metadata Key (AEMK) is derived from TEK using the computation $AEMK_i = HKDF(TEK_i, NULL, UTF8(\text{"EN-AEMK"}), 16)$. The Associated Encrypted Metadata (AEM) at a Unix Epoch Time j is derived from AEMK as per $AEM_{i,j} = AES\text{-}CTR128(AEMK_i, RPI_{i,j}, Metadata)$, where AES-CTR128 is AES-128 block cipher in counter mode. The metadata can be decrypted by the receiving app at a later point of time for additional verification only after a match occurs between a proximity identifier value computed from the diagnosis key and the corresponding received RPI value.

3.4.3.3 Framework API

The framework API contains the following broad set of primitives:

- **ENStatus:** This signifies the overall status of the Exposure Notification System (the allowed values are "active," "bluetoothOff," "disabled," "restricted," and "unknown")
- **ENAuthorizationStatus:** The authorization status can have values of "authorized," "notAuthorized," "restricted," and "unknown"
- **ENRiskScore:** The risk score value (unsigned 1-byte integer)
- **ENRiskLevel:** It's the estimated risk of user's exposure (unsigned 1-byte integer)

- **ENManager:** Exposure Notification manager class including its API methods
- Some more classes and their associated APIs that help in getting the summary list of exposures, setting the configuration parameters related to exposure detection service, retrieving additional details of exposure events, etc.

Our idea of describing the above primitives is not to present an exhaustive listing of the APIs but instead to build a high-level understanding of how the Apple-Google Exposure Notification protocol is structured into its various components and layers. This understanding would help us while doing system analysis.

3.4.4   Highlights and Characteristics

We now look at the highlights and characteristics of this specification.

It's the user who is in charge: One of the most prominent characteristics of the protocol and the framework is that it has weaved in user's consent at different stages of its operation. For the app to run properly, the user has to explicitly provide consent to enable the Exposure Notification Service in his/her device. The exposure risk level (or risk-score) is computed at the device end and if the user is diagnosed positive, it is only after he/she agrees the diagnosis keys from his/her device would get uploaded to the diagnosis server at the backend. The protocol does not require any personal or personally identifiable information of the user to run. Moreover, it can't be utilized by any app that requires access to geo-location of the user. Users may decide to stop using this functionality at any point of time by turning off the Exposure Notification Service or by uninstalling the contact tracing app (at which point all local data also gets deleted). In fact, this functionality of the protocol of not sharing exposure event details with the backend server pushed quite a few countries (like the United Kingdom) to move away from the Apple-Google framework in favour of creating home-grown centralized solutions.

Background mode of operation: This is undoubtedly the strongest feature of this protocol. While using ENF, the DCT app can transparently run in the background (both in Android and iOS platforms) and thereby consuming very less power and creating a hassle free user experience. There is no other protocol or system at this point that can boast of this functionality. Perhaps that is the main reason why this framework is getting adopted at a fast pace by a large number of countries and states [5] including, Canada (COVID Shield), Denmark (smittestop), Germany (Corona Warn), Italy (Immuni), Japan (COCOA), Poland (ProteGO Safe), Saudi Arabia (Tabaud), Spain (Radar COVID), Switzerland (SwissCovid), etc. as well as many states in the US.

Further integration at the OS level: Google and Apple have already integrated the service at the OS level in such a way that one may get the benefit of the functionality even in absence of a specific DCT app. It has also paved the way for multiple DCT apps that are based on this API framework to inter-operate.

Modular architecture: The entire framework has been developed in three layers—Bluetooth layer, Cryptography layer, and Framework API layer. This modularization not only helps the system to be used by multiple apps as per country-specific implementation, but any of the three layers can be easily customized and/or replaced if there is any such need. For example, if the device manufacturers come up with a physical communication protocol that is better than BLE, ENF may simply replace the Bluetooth layer of implementation with the new physical/link layer protocol. Similarly, if different cryptographic primitives are to be used for better security or faster computation, etc., the Cryptographic layer can be replaced with a new implementation. The apps would continue to function even if there happens to be any such change in the underlying layers.

3.4.5 System Analysis

We first present the security analysis and then concentrate upon the architecture analysis of the systems. We point out the possible open areas within each of these parts.

3.4.5.1 Security Analysis

The specifications corresponding to each layer (BLE, Cryptographic, and API) have already been outlined in the Protocol Details subsection. Hence, we directly get into the discussion of how the framework may respond to the different attack scenarios.

- **Backend impersonation:** Interestingly, the current protocol specification is entirely centered around the user-app. The backend implementations are left to be defined by the individual administrative authorities of the countries or states that decide to build their systems using the Exposure Notification Framework. Hence, the possibility of backend impersonation may not be ruled out and it would depend on the level of security and certification followed for the server that acts as the diagnosis key repository. A malicious backend server can cause harm in various ways (e.g., by sharing bogus diagnosis keys with the apps and thereby generating large scale False Negatives). To mitigate this attack the approval process of the app (from the designated app stores) must include checks and balances on the server certification, domain name registration, security protocol used in the communication channel between app and backend server, etc.
- **Server data breach:** Unless the country or state-specific implementation of the framework expects the user to share any personal or personally identifiable information at the time of registration, the backend server(s) would not have any such

sensitive data elements. Hence, in the event of data breach at the server end, there would be no serious risk of losing sensitive data. However, there exists a considerable risk of deanonymization of infected users who have uploaded their diagnosis keys to the server.

- **Replay attack:** This could be feasible within the 10-min time-interval of an epoch since the RPI value remains constant in such an interval. To bring further granularity of time interval beyond which Replay Attack can be neutralized, Associated Encrypted Metadata (AEM) field could be used to accommodate some kind of time-stamp as well.
- **Relay attack:** This attack is feasible.
- **Deanonymization of users:** Since the diagnosis keys of the infected users are directly downloaded by every user-app, deanonymization can be masterminded by malicious users or user groups. Such users may arrange to passively listen to RPIs of users (along with additional information like captured images of people who would have come near the RPI capturing devices), especially in places where the density of infected users is expected to be high (like in hospitals) and matching those against the RPIs generated from the diagnosis keys that are downloaded from the backend server. One-entry attack can also lead to deanonymization.
- **Inverse-Sybil attack:** Since the system does not verify the actual device or SIM card number to authenticate the messages between the app and the server, the inverse-Sybil attack is feasible.
- **Coercion threats:** An infected person's device can be misused by a malicious third party (before he/she uploads the proximity data to the server) by deliberately bringing that device in proximity to a large number of people and thereby triggering many false alarms in the ecosystem.
- **Miscellaneous:** The framework can be susceptible to Denial of Service (DoS) attack and many other generic mobile device's OS or API layer attacks.

3.4.5.2 Possible Open Areas

In the previous subsection, we have talked about the possible attacks to which the Exposure Notification Framework appears to be susceptible as per current specifications. In addition, there are certain areas of the protocol and the APIs that may require further investigation. These are as follows:

- There is no mention of message authentication at the BLE protocol layer. Hence, it is not clear how the framework recommends the handling of message tampering.
- The server to server communication across countries or states may need to be handled in an ad-hoc fashion. At this point, there is no uniform clear specification on how the backend servers may communicate with each other in a federated system where multiple states of a country (e.g., the USA) may go for different implementations while following the same framework as in such a case there would be a need for people to move across state borders without losing the benefit of the system.

In Sect. 3.4.4, we have covered architectural elements. We now describe some of the possible open areas.

- There are insufficient details on how ENF expects the user registration process to happen. If a user's app crashes and the user registers afresh to the system after installing the app again, would the previous user-id be linkable to the new user-id? If not, would the previous history of exposure be lost forever?
- The calibration of signal strengths for different manufacturers' devices in the broadcast topology can be a critical success factor for the system to be effective—the calibration process (or any reference signal strength data) has not been shared along with the specification.
- The specifications talk about metadata like signal strength or duration being used in the risk-scoring algorithm, but it has not elaborated on how that would be captured.

3.5 East Coast PACT

East Coast PACT (Private Automated Contact Tracing) protocol has been jointly developed by Massachusetts Institute of Technology's (MIT's) Computer Science and Artificial Intelligence Laboratory (CSAIL), Massachusetts General Hospital Center for Global Health, MIT Internet Policy Research Initiative, MIT Lincoln Laboratory with additional collaborators including MIT Media Lab, Boston University, Brown University, Carnegie Mellon University, the Weizmann Institute, and other R&D centers. We refer to Version 0.1 of the protocol specification [25] that got released on 8 April 2020 and the Mission and Approach document [27] for our discussion. As per the PACT team, their protocol is largely similar to the Apple-Google Exposure Notification Framework, DP3T, and TCN proposals. It is licensed under the Creative Commons Attribution 4.0 License.

3.5.1 Framework and Protocol Details

In this framework, there are primarily two protocol layers—(1) the chirping layer and (2) the tracing layer. We now describe the protocols for both the layers.

Chirping Layer: The proximity identifiers (referred as "chirps") are 28 bytes long and these are generated from certain "seed values." The seed values (which are random 32-byte values) are generated every hour and stored in the device along with the current time. If r_t denotes the chirp value at time t (measured to a precision of 1 min), and s is the seed value in that hour, then $r_t = \mathrm{PRF}(s, t)$, where PRF is a pseudorandom function. The chirps are sent every few seconds over the BLE interface to nearby devices in broadcast topology mode.

When a device receives a chirp from another device, it stores the same in the "contact log" along with additional information of signal strength and location-specific information (optionally). The time is measured in this protocol with a 1-min precision and therefore if multiple chirps are received from a device within a minute, only one such chirp and the maximum signal strength (as a proxy for the distance between the devices) would be stored. The protocol also expects every implemented system to store the seed values corresponding to the chirp values sent by the device along with the time when it was sent. The specification recommends keeping the logs in the device for 3 months. It must be noted that when chirps are sent, no metadata is attached along with that value. As per the current specification, there is no provision to store additional information—like whether the other person is wearing a mask or any protective gear, the type of location (e.g., open space or closed space), etc., in the contact log.

Tracing Layer: This layer helps a user-app to determine the risk-score of getting infected. Whenever a user is diagnosed positive by a diagnostic center, a valid permission number (that may be used only once) is given by the test center to the user which would allow him/her to upload the seeds to a backend server (& database) corresponding to the chirps that his/her app have been sending over a period of time for which the user could have been contagious. The uploading of seeds instead of chirp values helps in optimizing the size of the transmitted data to the backend server. The upload format follows a tuple structure like (s, t_1, t_2), where t_1 and t_2 signify the start and end time of the hour for which the seed was valid. The choice of upload lies with the user and even during the uploading process, the user may decide not to upload the seed values of certain hours due to privacy reasons in which case the app would allow the user to redact certain entries by generating fresh random numbers for those durations.

To check if the user is at risk of being infected, the user-app can download the exposure database (in case the database is geographically divided, only a part of the database may need to be downloaded), generate the chirp values corresponding to the seed values, cross-check the chirp values with its contact log to see if there is any match and if the time-window is approximately the same. The number of matches with chirp values generated from a particular seed value would reveal the duration of the event and the metadata of signal strength may reveal the average distance between the two devices. These data points are important to detect possible contact events where the user could have been exposed to other users who have been diagnosed positive later. The number of such contact events together can be used to derive a risk-score and, at this stage, there is a possibility of also exposing the granular details about the contact events to the user. The specification advises that users eventually need to consult medical professionals who can decide based on the risk-score and other data points (like user's health condition, symptoms, location, etc.) and recommend the appropriate next steps to the user.

The specification has also considered the possibility of implementing chirp repeaters with a delay to handle the surface transmissions. For different reasons (e.g., for spotting the concentration zones and the nature of spread of the disease) if the location needs to be stored as metadata in the chirps, the protocol suggests a mechanism through which it may remain encrypted in the local device storage with keys derived from the seed values of the contacts and therefore the deciphering would be feasible only for the matched entries and for no other cases.

3.5.2   Highlights

3.5.2.1   The PACT Initiative

The PACT team has embarked on four major lines of effort:

- Proximity detection efficacy: Experimenting and objectively evaluating the BLE performance to determine the criteria for two devices to be "Too Close For Too Long (TC4TL)" as per epidemiological and medical guidelines and sharing the gathered results and insights with Public Health Authorities (PHA), with Apple-Google team and other teams for better decision making. The PACT team also plans to start investigating other signaling technologies (e.g., ultrasound, UWB, etc.)
- Privacy: Assess privacy impact of the integration of digital contact tracing systems with public health systems, study the developments of Apple-Google framework and gather insights with respect to the actual experience of users vs privacy-preserving goals of these systems.
- Integration: System architecture study of integrating multiple systems across geographical regions and advising Public Health Authorities based on the findings.
- Public health efficacy: To study how these systems can bolster the efforts of manual contact tracing and show measurable progress of controlling the pandemic over time.

The PACT stack is divided into three parts and it has focused on addressing challenges related to each of the parts separately.

- Layer 1: Proximity measurement
- Layer 2: Private cryptographic protocol
- Layer 3: (a) Public health interface and (b) Individual interface

The PACT team is focused on cross-layer activities that include

- Prototype building
- System analysis
- Data collection and experimentation
- Develop and roll out pilots for select organizations

3.5.3   Design Principles

- Designed with simplicity of understanding and implementation in mind
- Compatibility with other decentralized protocols have also been a key factor of the specification

- It has been designed with the principles of autonomy, openness, and transparency (including the measures of graceful "sunset" at the end of the pandemic) and to uphold the values of user's privacy and civil liberties without compromising the social health issues
- The size and rate of chirps have been designed in such a way that a wide range of device/OS combinations can be handled
- It can be easily integrated with Apple Find My protocol.

3.5.4 System Analysis

The system analysis of this protocol has a considerable overlap with the system analysis of the Apple-Google framework—hence we refer to the same in most of the places.

3.5.4.1 Security Analysis

We directly get into the discussion of how the framework may respond to the different attack scenarios.

- **Backend impersonation:** This would be identical to the analysis presented in case of Apple-Google framework.
- **Server data breach:** This would be similar to the analysis presented in case of Apple-Google framework, except here the seed values allow generation of all the chirps that have been emitted in an hour and hence the possibility of deanonymization of some of the infected users or creation of contact graphs corresponding to such users would be even more.
- **Replay attack:** This could be feasible within the 1 min time-interval within which the chirp value remains constant.
- **Relay attack:** This attack is feasible.
- **Deanonymization of users:** Since the seed values of the infected users are directly downloaded by every user-app, deanonymization can be masterminded by malicious users or user groups in a way similar to the attack described in case of Apple-Google framework. One-entry attack can also lead to deanonymization.
- **Inverse-Sybil attack:** Possible. This would be identical to the analysis presented in case of Apple-Google framework.
- **Coercion threats:** Possible. This would be identical to the analysis presented in case of Apple-Google framework.
- **Address carryover attacks:** This is possible as nothing has been mentioned of how to prevent the same in BLE layer.
- **Miscellaneous:** Possible. This would be identical to the analysis presented in case of Apple-Google framework.

3.5.4.2   Possible Open Areas

Apart from the vulnerabilities to the attacks mentioned in the previous subsection, the additional open areas of the protocol are as follows.

- The distinction between the responsibilities of different layers (API layer, cryptographic layer, and BLE layer) has not been mentioned.
- The details about the actual cryptographic/coding primitives and algorithms used have not been included.
- There is no mention of message authentication at the BLE protocol layer. Hence, it is not clear how the framework recommends the handling of message tampering.
- There is no clear specification on how the backends may communicate with each other in a federated system of servers.

The possible open areas in architectural description need to be enumerated too.

- The user registration process has not been described.
- The fault tolerance aspect of the framework at device end or server end has not been outlined.
- The calibration of signal strengths for different manufacturers' devices in the broadcast topology can be a critical success factor for the system to be effective—the calibration process (or any reference signal strength data) has not been shared along with the specification.
- The specifications talk about metadata like signal strength or duration being used in the risk-scoring algorithm, but it has not elaborated on how that would be captured.

Next, we concentrate on West Coast PACT.

3.6   West Coast PACT

Privacy-Sensitive Protocols And Mechanisms for Mobile Contact Tracing (PACT) is a protocol that has been proposed by a team of technologists and researchers associated with the Paul G. Allen School of Computer Science and Engineering, University of Washington Medicine and Microsoft, through a white paper [28] published on 7 April 2020. The corresponding Github repository [8] contains a reference implementation of the same. As noted in the East Coast PACT specification document [25] that there are a lot of similarities in the approach and structure between the two proposals.

3.6.1   Framework and Protocol Details

One important element, that is different in the framework as compared to other decentralized systems, is that it allows the seeds of the infected users to be either published by the hospitals post their validation and confirmation or alternatively self-reported by the users who are diagnosed as positive. We now describe the protocol design in brief.

There are two basic parameters—a number Δ and a unit of time dt such that $\Delta \cdot dt$ (product) equals the infection window as guided by the epidemiologists (which could be typically 2 weeks). The pseudorandom IDs that are emitted by a device are 128-bit long. The ith ID (ID_i) is broadcast during the ith time-window where the first time-window is assumed to have started from the time the user-app got initialized (say t_0). The protocol samples an initial 128-bit seed (called S_0) and each successive seed (S_{i+1}) as well as the successive pseudorandom ID (ID_{i+1}) is generated using the following step

$$(S_{i+1}, ID_{i+1}) \leftarrow G(S_i),$$

where G is a cryptographic pseudorandom generator using a hash function SHA-256. The first ID is ID_1, as the entire procedure starts with S_0. When a device receives a pseudo-random ID from a neighboring device, the app stores it in the local storage with a time-stamp as a pair (ID, t). At the time of reporting, the infected user needs to upload the seed value (S^*) that corresponds to the time-window at the start of the infectious period (2 weeks back), the starting time (t_{start}), and the ending time (t_{end}). This tuple gets added to the list of exposed seed values in the public server. These entries can be validated by attaching signature σ and (optionally) a certificate ($cert$).

To check exposure, a user-app needs to download all such exposed seed value tuples, derive the corresponding ID-values for the durations indicated in the tuples, check for any matching with the local storage of received IDs, and compute the risk of exposure. The time-stamps are used for validation of the possible exposure events (e.g., to prevent relay attacks).

3.6.2 Highlights

The protocol minimizes the information a user needs to share with the central server. The users cannot upload any information to the server (before being or) once outside the infection period. It recommends that the app should upload the infection information to the central server with a slight time delay, which helps in reducing the chances of replay attacks. The protocol also prevents leakage of information regarding the app-joining date by fixing the length of the ID-sequence to a value Δ. Additionally, strong integrity of the server data can be added to the existing mechanism by introducing an authentication-verification process to the uploading procedure using a pair of keys (sk, vk).

The white paper [28] discusses the ease of interoperability of decentralized protocols similar to East Coast PACT, West Coast PACT, and DP3T due to the same basic principle of uploading seeds to a server. However, it also points out that the only difficulty that may arise is due to differences in the reliability of privacy-protection of users uploading this data. This can be addressed by introducing a common API.

The ethics of achieving a balance between the privacy of users and transferring information to the authorities in the interest of safety of the larger population are also discussed. These considerations are likely to differ greatly between different countries. Finally, the accessibility of these services depends most importantly on the number of people owning a smartphone and installing the app, which greatly affects their effectiveness.

3.6.3   System Analysis

The system analysis of this protocol is almost identical to that of East Coast PACT due to the similarity between the two proposals.

3.6.3.1   Security Analysis

- **Backend impersonation:** Possible and identical to the situation as in East Coast PACT or Apple-Google Framework.
- **Server data breach:** The risk and extent of deanonymization in this system are much more than that of any other decentralized protocols since here the starting seed value (S^*) is sufficient to generate all the ID values that have been broadcast by the infected user's app within the window of infection. There is no other risk of disclosure as no personal or personally identifiable information of users gets stored in the public server.
- **Replay attack:** This could be feasible for the dt time-interval within which the broadcast ID values remain constant.
- **Relay attack:** This attack is feasible.
- **Deanonymization of users:** The risk and extent of deanonymization in this system are much more than that of any other decentralized protocols since here the starting seed value (S^*) is sufficient to generate all the ID values that have been broadcast by the infected user's app within the window of infection. This weakness also risks other data such as time of exposure or location of the infected user to be released. The possible mitigation provided in [38] involves only releasing the IDs and not seeds from the uploaded data, which still does not prevent dedicated adversaries from establishing a link.
- **Inverse-Sybil attack:** Possible and identical to the situation as in East Coast PACT or Apple-Google Framework.
- **Coercion threats:** This would be identical to the situation as in case of East Coast PACT or Apple-Google framework.
- **Address carryover attacks:** This is possible as nothing has been mentioned of how to prevent the same in BLE layer.
- **Miscellaneous:** Same as in East Coast PACT or Apple-Google framework.

3.6.3.2 Possible Open Areas

Apart from the vulnerabilities to the attacks mentioned in the previous subsection, the additional open areas of the protocol are as follows.

- The distinction between the responsibilities of different layers (API layer, cryptographic layer, and BLE layer) have not been mentioned. The specification does not provide the details of how to configure and use the BLE layer and how to make it compatible with different platforms and device manufacturers.
- Although the specification talks about the need for a common API to ensure interoperability among multiple decentralized systems, the mechanism of interoperability between multiple public servers using the same protocol for different states/countries or the details of the common API have not been described.

There are also certain open areas in architecture.

- The user registration process has not been described.
- The fault tolerance aspect of the framework at device end or server end has not been outlined.
- The specification does not outline the risk-scoring algorithm. It also does not specify the way to calibrate the signals emitted by the devices which can be used as a proxy to measure the approximate distance between two nearby devices (e.g., in the specification it talks about a distance of 6m to be used as the expected proximity).

3.6.4 A Re-Randomized Version

The authors of [28] have also proposed an alternative dual approach, where infected users, on authorization from the health authority, upload to the server not their broadcasted identifiers, but the received ones. A small advantage gained in this dual approach is the restriction of deanonymization and linkage attacks by the server if the received identifiers are uploaded in an encrypted form. However, it becomes very easy for malicious users to achieve replay, relay, inverse-Sybil, and deanonymization attacks in this case (say C comes into contact with B and sends the received identifiers to A for upload when A is diagnosed positive). The broadcast and upload of identifiers are proposed to be executed through the decisional Diffie-Hellman (DDH) protocol, by choosing a cyclic group G with a generator g known to all entities, and each user choosing one's own secret key s_U. On contact with another user B, the device of user A receives and stores the pair $(g^{r_i}, g^{r_i \cdot s_B})$. On positive diagnosis, A gets authentication from the health authority and uploads all pairs (x, y) received from such contacts to the server.

A possible mitigation for deanonymization attacks is for A to choose a random element $r \in G$ and upload (x^r, y^r) to the server instead of the received values. A user B wanting to know one's risk status can simply check whether $x^{s_B} = y$ for any of the pairs downloaded from the server. This would prevent B from deanonymizing A in spite of (say) recording data such as a list of one's contacts at the time the particular identifier was being broadcasted.

3.7 Temporary Contact Numbers (TCN)

Temporary Contact Number (TCN) is one of the earliest decentralized protocols that was introduced [9] on March 17 2020 by a group of researchers, engineers, private and public health experts through a collaborative effort between Stanford University and the University of Waterloo. It has been developed by the TCN coalition that includes the Covid Watch [7] and the CoEpi [4] teams. The updated version of the specification and its corresponding open-source reference implementation is available in the Github repository [32].

3.7.1 Framework and Protocol Details

Since there is a lot of similarity of TCN with the previously described systems like Apple-Google Framework, DP3T, East Coast PACT, and West Coast PACT, we would present it at a high level by primarily highlighting the specific features that are not observed in the other decentralized protocols.

Here, the proximity identifiers, referred as the Temporary Contact Numbers (TCNs), are generated as 128-bit pseudonymous pseudorandom numbers (at the device end) from a seed value. Like the rest of the decentralized systems, the reason for using the seed values for generating the TCNs, in contrast to the direct genera-tion of pseudorandom numbers, is to optimize the size of data upload at the time of reporting (by users who are later diagnosed positive). We now describe the details of the steps through which the TCNs get generated.

At first, a pair of keys, called the Report Authorization Key (RAK) and the Report Verification Key (RVK) get generated using the Ed25519 signature scheme [21]. An initial Temporary Contact Key (TCK_0) is created using a SHA-256 hash function (called H_TCK), where $\text{TCK}_0 = \text{H\_TCK(RAK)}$. This initial TCK is used to generate a series of TCKs ($\text{TCK}_1, \text{TCK}_2, \ldots$, etc.) which in turn generate a series of TCN values ($\text{TCN}_1, \text{TCN}_2, \ldots$, etc.) using another SHA-256 hash function (called H_TCN).

$$\text{TCK}_i = \text{H\_TCK}(\text{RVK} \,||\, \text{TCK}_{i-1}) \text{ and}$$
$$\text{TCN}_i = \text{H\_TCN}(\text{le\_u16}(i) \,||\, \text{TCK}_i) \text{ for every integral } i > 0.$$

The report generation process is extremely compact in TCN. The core idea comes from the observation that if RVK and a starting TCK value is provided along with the index values that correspond to the starting and ending TCN values, the receiving user-app can easily derive all the required TCNs. The specific details are now given below.

$$\text{REPORT} = (\text{RVK} \parallel \text{le\_u16}(s) \parallel \text{le\_u}(e) \parallel \text{memo}) \text{ and}$$
$$\text{SIGNED\_REPORT} = \text{REPORT} \parallel \text{SIG}$$

In the above calculations, s and e are the starting and ending indices (corresponding to the epochs within which the user is considered to be infectious and usually this period is considered to be 14 days), 'memo' is a free-form implementation specific message (of the form TAG ‖ LENGTH_OF(DATA) ‖ DATA) and SIG is the signature on the REPORT (based on RAK) that would serve the purpose of authentication.

The specification has mentioned that a user-app should download the signed seed reports of the infected users on a daily basis from the server and evaluate the extent of exposure of the corresponding user.

The "encounter handshake" part of the protocol between the devices is implemented in both broadcast topology as well as through connected topology so that Android and iOS-based devices (running in either foreground or background mode) can be supported. The "infection reporting" part of the protocol is implemented using a secured HTTPS channel.

3.7.2 Highlights

- Like the rest of the decentralized protocols, no personally identifiable information is required at any stage for the protocol to function
- The protocol can work with either verified test results or self-reported symptoms
- Typically a signed report would be 134–389 bytes long
- The pair of keys RAK and RVK should be periodically rotated so that the TCN history does not form a single long reproducible chain. However, if it changes too soon, the scalability of the protocol may get impacted. In that case, the report upload also should be done in separate chunks and the specification has suggested a duration of not more than 6 h for every report.
- The design of the protocol has kept in mind the following needs:

  - Cross User-app and cross-platform (iOS and Android) device interaction
  - Not asking the user for location access from his/her device
  - Efficient usage of BLE power
  - Workability even in the background mode of the app
  - The duration for which one TCN value remains constant is a configurable parameter. It is recommended that it should be aligned with the change of MAC value as well to avoid linkage attacks—however, the specification has pointed out that the current implementation is not guaranteed to achieve that in Android or iOS due to the inherent issues of the operating systems.

3.7.3 Security and Architecture Analysis

- **Backend impersonation:** Like most of the decentralized protocols (like Apple-Google Framework, DP3T, East Coast PACT, etc.) TCN is also susceptible to this attack.
- **Server data breach:** Susceptible to this attack in a way similar to East Coast PACT.
- **Replay attack:** Susceptible to this attack in a way similar to East Coast PACT.
- **Relay attack:** This attack is feasible.
- **Deanonymization of users:** Susceptible to this attack in a way similar to East Coast PACT.
- **Inverse-Sybil attack:** Like most of the decentralized protocols (like Apple-Google Framework, DP3T, East Coast PACT, etc.) TCN is also susceptible to this attack.
- **Coercion threats:** Like most of the decentralized protocols (like Apple-Google Framework, DP3T, East Coast PACT, etc.) TCN is also susceptible to this attack.
- **Address and Shared Carryover Attacks:** TCN is susceptible to both these attacks and the specification has also talked about these possibilities.
- **Miscellaneous:** Possible. This would be identical to the analysis presented in case of Apple-Google framework.

3.7.3.1 Possible Open Areas in Security

Apart from the vulnerabilities to the attacks mentioned in the previous subsection, the additional open areas of the protocol are as follows.

- The distinction between the responsibilities of different layers (API layer, cryptographic layer, and BLE layer) has not been mentioned.
- There is no clear specification on how the backends may communicate with each other in a federated system of servers.
- There is a significant detailing done for cross-platform usage. However, no guidelines or experience sharing has been done for cross-app usage.
- The validation of reporting stage through Health Authority has not been explained enough

3.7.3.2 Possible Open Areas in Architecture

- The user registration process has not been described.
- The fault tolerance aspect of the framework at device end or server end has not been outlined.
- The calibration of signal strengths for different manufacturers' devices in the broadcast topology can be a critical success factor for the system to be effective—the calibration process (or any reference signal strength data) has not been shared along with the specification.

- There is no mention of how epidemiologists may get help from the system by tracking the progress of the disease, its transmission mechanism, or the dynamic nature of spread of infection across multiple locations.

3.8 The Epione Protocol

A team of researchers from UC Berkeley and the National University of Singapore has proposed the **Epione** protocol [36] for contact tracing and preventing the spread of SARS-CoV-2. The *registration phase* of this protocol begins with users installing the app and generating random tokens using a secret key κ, which are broadcast through Bluetooth in the *contact-broadcast phase*. Users store the received tokens on a local list on their devices. The health authority is considered to be a trusted entity and is responsible for identifying infected users and reporting the PRG seeds used to generate their broadcasted tokens to the server. The seeds are forwarded by the infected users to the health authority after encryption using a public key pk (of a public key-secret key pair (pk, sk) generated by the server), which the health authority forwards to the server. The server is also trusted and can decrypt these seeds using its secret key, and use them to generate and store the broadcasted tokens in a (private) list. This constitutes the *reporting phase* of the Epione protocol, after which, the *exposure calculation phase* can take place when a user and the server securely compare the user's received tokens with the list of tokens broadcasted by infected users stored on the server with a matching algorithm (that uses a secure two-party private set intersection cardinality (PSI-CA) computation). Although the central server has access to all the tokens received by any user, it is difficult for it to compute the neighborhood of any infected user (considered as a vertex of the proximity graph) due to the unavailability of tokens received by undiagnosed users. Therefore, Epione is a decentralized contact tracing protocol according to our classification.

3.8.1 Private Set Intersection (PSI)

Epione uses a secure two-party private set intersection cardinality (PSI-CA) computation to assess the risk exposure of querying users, by determining the size of the intersection set of two lists, one containing the tokens broadcasted by infected users saved in the server database, and another containing the tokens received by a user queried to the server. A user wanting to know one's risk has full access to one's own list but does not have direct access to the list stored on the server. The server, on the other hand, does not have direct access to the tokens received by the querying user. Algorithms that compute information about the intersection of two sets without complete knowledge of the elements in at least one of the two sets are called *private set intersection (PSI)* algorithms.

PSI algorithms could be of different types, based on the information computed about the intersecting set. These types range from computing the complete intersection to only finding the size of the intersection to simply stating whether intersection occurs or not. Suppose A has a set $\{x_1, \ldots, x_n\}$ and B has a set $\{y_1, \ldots, y_m\}$, which they do not wish to fully reveal to each other. The simplest way to find the intersection between these two sets is to apply a variation of the Diffie-Hellman key-exchange protocol on each element of both the sets [23]. A and B agree on a hash function H (but do not share the hash key they choose). A chooses an element a belonging to the underlying field and computes $\{H(x_1)^a, \ldots, H(x_n)^a\}$, while B chooses an element b and computes $\{H(y_1)^b, \ldots, H(y_m)^b\}$. They exchange these lists, compute $\{H(y_1)^{ab}, \ldots, H(y_m)^{ab}\}$ and $\{H(x_1)^{ab}, \ldots, H(x_n)^{ab}\}$ respectively and again exchange these two lists.

If each participant randomly permutes one's list in both the exchanges, then they only know the size of the intersection. If the lists are randomly permuted only in the first exchange, they would know the positions of the elements that are present in the intersection set but not their values. If the lists are randomly permuted in the second exchange, they would know the exact values that are common in both the lists. All these cases are subject to the collision properties of the hash function H, which, if not used, would directly reveal the complete sets to both participants.

The particular case of revealing only the size of the intersection set is called a *private set intersection cardinality (PSI-CA)* algorithm.

3.8.2 Highlights of the Epione Protocol

Epione stands out from centralized protocols through the token generation process, which takes place locally on the user-apps. The tokens received from other users are also stored locally on the users' devices. However, it is also different from decentralized protocols due to the absence of any bulletin board maintenance by the server. Instead, users query their received tokens to the server, which computes their exposure risks. Since it implements the token-matching algorithm through a PSI-CA computation, the server only gains knowledge of the size of the intersection of the set of received token queried by a user and the set of tokens of infected users reported by the health authorities. This prevents the server from gaining information about any particular user, thus restricting a neighborhood-construction of any infected user in the proximity graph. It seems to be satisfactorily secure against most semi-honest adversaries.

3.8.3 Possible Cryptographic Issues with the Epione Protocol

Although this system may prevent attacks from malicious users (and possibly other non-user, non-authority entities) due to centralization, it places complete trust in the health authority and partial trust in the central server. A corrupted health authority may quite easily carry out attacks involving false-positive claims. A server colluding with the health authority equipped with only a weakly secure implementation of a PSI-CA computation for its matching algorithm could also carry out (possibly) complete linkage attacks. These attacks have been mitigated in [36] by stressing on the trustworthiness of these two entities and on the requirement of not allowing them to collude.

Malicious adversaries with abilities to intercept or read various transmitted data could also launch quite strong attacks on the system. For example, if an adversary gains access to the communication between a group of users querying their received tokens to the server and the server's corresponding answers, it could work out at least an incomplete neighborhood of infected users whose tokens were shared with multiple users of this group. Such an adversary might also track users to a large extent. Arbitrary queries by malicious adversaries have been proposed to be mitigated by use of a cryptographic hash on the tokens queried, although it must be noted that this is not a feature of the original system proposed.

3.9 An Approach to Avoid Inverse-Sybil Attacks

The work [34] proposes an interesting protocol to avoid attacks on these protocols similar in nature to inverse-Sybil attacks. It makes use of three hash functions and requires each user to maintain a hash-chain to validate one's uploaded identifiers. The first two stages of the protocol are divided into epochs, at the start of which, the process begins afresh. After registration, the *setup phase* begins when each user chooses a hash key k and a starting (current) hash-chain head value h. The first hash function, H_1 is used to generate subsequent hash-chain heads for each epoch. Next, the *broadcast phase* includes the following steps. When an epoch starts, a user samples a random value and broadcasts it along with the current hash-chain head. A user also receives such pairs from any other users in one's vicinity. The received random values are stored in a set C, which is constructed by hashing the triple of the user's current hash head, the received hash head and the received random value by means of the second hash function H_2, and the sent random values are stored in an evaluation list (L^{eval}) by hashing the triple of the received hash head, the user's current hash head and the sent random value by means of the third hash function H_3. A report list (L^{rep}) is created by recording pairs of each set C and the corresponding hash-chain head, which, in addition to the user's hash key k, would be reported to the server in the *reporting phase* if the user is tested positive for SARS-CoV-2. The server only proceeds if it can check that the hash-chain heads in the report list uploaded by a user indeed form a hash-chain. In this case, it stores the hashed values $H_3(h_i, \sigma)$, for each $\sigma \in C_i$, for each $(h_i, C_i) \in L^{\text{rep}}$, in the server list ($L^{\text{ser}}$). In the *exposure calculation phase*, a user wanting to check one's exposure status can download (the full or a part of) L^{ser} and check whether any entries match with its L^{eval}. The user is considered at risk if any such matches exist.

This is clearly a non-interactive decentralized protocol as users need not interact with echo other on coming into contact and the only broadcast of identifiers suffices, and since the central server does not get any information about the contacts of infected users and therefore cannot (honestly) construct their proximity graphs. A second protocol, which is decentralized and instead uses location data for chaining is also discussed in [34]. It is very similar to the one described here, but instead of simply storing hashed values of the hash-chain heads and random values broadcasted or received, a user's location and time coordinates are also stored in the L^{rep} and L^{eval} lists on the device. This may cause loss of privacy (depending upon the security of the hash functions), but increases the integrity of the system, further tightening security against inverse-Sybil, replay, and relay attacks.

3.10   Conclusion

The decentralized contact tracing protocols discussed here all share key elements such as the minimization of information that a user needs to share with the central server, this uploading of information being a voluntary action that a user may take only on testing positive for SARS-CoV-2, and in no other case. The server broadcasts this information in a manner that maintains the anonymity of all infected users who have uploaded their IDs, for only the time period that these users may be deemed infectious. These users also cannot upload any information to the server (before being or) once outside the infection period. A user wanting to check one's status of exposure need not share any information with the server at all and can compute this risk locally on the app.

All these protocols may eventually allow interoperability between different apps due to the similarity in their approaches. However, it must be noted that difficulties may arise due to differences in the reliability of privacy-protection of users uploading this data. This can be addressed by introducing a common API. Some unavoidable issues such as immediate identification of an infected user (say A) by another user (say B), if A is the only user to have established contact with B, are present in the systems. There is complete privacy for users who have not tested positive for SARS-CoV-2, but some privacy loss occurs whenever a user uploads one's keys or identifiers to the server.

It may be worthwhile to expand the current scope of these systems by considering ways to perform contact tracing (with explicit approval from users) to secondary and tertiary levels and have a much broader view of the spread by analyzing the secondary or tertiary proximity graphs combined with the compartmental model of the infection system dynamics used by epidemiologists. Another question to ponder is the extension of the system's functionality from a human-to-human transmission alerting function to flagging potential infectious-surface-to-human transmission events (the possible third way of transmission through aerosol particles may not be feasible to be captured by the current level of technology). It may also be worthwhile to investigate possible alternate implementations of the systems that do not require BLE or the extension of some of the functionalities in feature phones as well. Furthermore, a user may want to perform certain "what-if" analyses of routes (combined with the GPS location map app) to get an apriori idea of the risk involved in traveling on a specific route. It would be of interest to inspect whether this information can be provided to some extent, with extreme caution, as it would decrease the privacy provisions of the system, despite its usefulness. Finally, the accessibility of these services depends most importantly on the number of people owning a smartphone and installing the app, which would greatly affect their effectiveness.

References

1. Apple-Google. Privacy-preserving contact tracing. https://www.apple.com/covid19/contacttracing.
2. Apple-Google. Privacy-preserving contact tracing. Exposure notification FAQs. https://blog.google/documents/73/Exposure_Notification_-_FAQ_v1.1.pdf.
3. Castelluccia, C., Bielova, N., Boutet, A., Cunche, M., Lauradoux, C., Le Métayer, D., Roca, V. (2020). DESIRE: A third way for a european exposure notification system leveraging the best of centralized and decentralized systems. ffhal-02570382 https://hal.inria.fr/hal-02570382/document.
4. CoEpi Website. https://www.coepi.org/about/.
5. COVID-19 Apps Wikipedia Page. https://en.wikipedia.org/wiki/COVID-19_apps.
6. COVIDSafe app. https://www.health.gov.au/resources/apps-and-tools/covidsafe-app.
7. COVIDWatch Wikipedia Page. https://en.wikipedia.org/wiki/Covid_Watch.
8. COVIDSafe. https://github.com/covidsafe.
9. CovidWatch Article. https://www.covid-watch.org/article/.
10. CovidWatch Website. https://www.covid-watch.org/.
11. DP3T Whitepaper. https://github.com/DP-3T/documents/blob/master/DP3T%20White%20Paper.pdf.
12. DP3T – Aims. https://github.com/DP-3T/documents/blob/master/DP3T%20-%20Aims%20of%20the%20Project.pdf.
13. DP3T – Overview document. https://github.com/DP-3T/documents/blob/master/DP3T%20-%20Simplified%20Three%20Page%20Brief.pdf.
14. DP3T Documents. https://github.com/DP-3T/documents.
15. DP3T Android App. https://github.com/DP-3T/dp3t-app-android-ch.
16. DP3T iOS App. https://github.com/DP-3T/dp3t-app-ios-ch.
17. DP3T - Interoperability decentralized proximity tracing specification (Preview). https://github.com/DP-3T/documents/blob/master/DP3T%20-%20Interoperability%20Decentralized%20Proximity%20Tracing%20Specification%20(Preview).pdf.
18. DP3T - Security analysis. https://github.com/DP-3T/documents/blob/master/Security%20analysis/Privacy%20and%20Security%20Attacks%20on%20Digital%20Proximity%20Tracing%20Systems.pdf.
19. DP3T - Authorization analysis. https://github.com/DP-3T/documents/blob/master/DP3T%20-%20Upload%20Authorisation%20Analysis%20and%20Guidelines.pdf.
20. DP3T - Exposure score calculation. https://github.com/DP-3T/documents/blob/master/DP3T%20-%20Exposure%20Score%20Calculation.pdf.
21. Edwards-curve digital signature algorithm (EdDSA) – Wikipedia Page, Subheading Ed25519. https://en.wikipedia.org/wiki/EdDSA#Ed25519.
22. Exposure Notification – Wiki. https://en.wikipedia.org/wiki/Exposure_Notification.

23. Huberman, B. A., Franklin, M., Hogg, T. (1999). Enhancing privacy and trust in electronic communities. In *EC '99: Proceedings of the 1st ACM conference on Electronic commerce. November 1999* (pp. 78–86). https://doi.org/10.1145/336992.337012.
24. Issues raised in GitHub repository for DP-3T. https://github.com/DP-3T/documents/issues.
25. PACT protocol specification - version 0.1 (4/8/2020) https://pact.mit.edu/wp-content/uploads/2020/04/The-PACT-protocol-specification-ver-0.1.pdf.
26. PACT MIT Webpage. https://pact.mit.edu/.
27. PACT – Mission and approach. https://pact.mit.edu/wp-content/uploads/2020/05/PACT-Mission-and-Approach-2020-05-19-.pdf.
28. PACT: Privacy-sensitive protocols and mechanisms for mobile contact tracing. https://arxiv.org/abs/2004.03544.
29. Pietrzak, K. Delayed authentication replay and relay attacks on DP-3T. https://eprint.iacr.org/2020/418.pdf.
30. ROBERT: ROBust and privacy-presERving proximity Tracing. Inria, France and Fraunhofer AISEC, Germany. https://github.com/ROBERT-proximity-tracing/documents.
31. Statement on the processing of personal data in the context of the COVID-19 outbreak – European Data Protection Board. https://edpb.europa.eu/sites/edpb/files/files/file1/edpb_statement_2020_processingpersonaldataandcovid-19_en.pdf.
32. Specification and reference implementation of the TCN Protocol for decentralized, privacy-preserving contact tracing. https://github.com/TCNCoalition/TCN.
33. Techcrunch.com News Article. Apple and Google release sample code, UI and detailed policies for COVID-19 exposure-notification apps. https://techcrunch.com/2020/05/04/apple-and-google-release-sample-code-and-detailed-policies-for-covid-19-exposure-notification-apps/.
34. The Crypto Group at IST Austria. Inverse-Sybil attacks in automated contact tracing. https://eprint.iacr.org/2020/670.
35. TraceTogether Wikipedia Page. https://en.wikipedia.org/wiki/TraceTogether.
36. Trieu, N., Shehata, K., Saxena, P., Shokri, R., Song, D. Epione: Lightweight contact tracing with strong privacy. arXiv:2004.13293.
37. Vaudenay, S. Centralized or decentralized? The contact tracing dilemma. https://eprint.iacr.org/2020/531.
38. Vaudenay, S. Analysis of DP-3T between scylla and charybdis. https://eprint.iacr.org/2020/399.pdf.

Chapter 4
Outline of a Proposal and Conclusion

Abstract In this chapter, we discuss the future of digital contact tracing systems and the evolving role of cryptography in this regard. We mostly concentrate on how a decentralized system should be designed maintaining the privacy of the users. We first consider an ideal system and then move forward towards a more realistic one. The assumptions and cryptologic issues are explained. The system may also be used as a centralized one with certain design modifications. We discuss higher order contact tracing in terms of the neighborhood of a neighborhood, i.e., one more level of indirection. This is the concluding chapter of this brief manuscript.

4.1 Lessons from the Past

Over a hundred years ago when the world reeled under the Spanish flu pandemic, there were no smartphones or even mobile phones, but manual contact tracing was used as one of the measures to contain and control the spread of the infection. While there has been a tremendous advancement of technology from the days of Spanish Flu to the present days of COVID-19, including the re-emergence of Artificial Intelligence (AI) from its long hibernation to a state where experts declared that AI is the new electricity [1] or that the singularity is near [5], it failed to either predict or make humanity ready for the current catastrophe. So we must go back and take a look at the history of epidemics, understand the complex issues around the age-old epidemiological tools like contact tracing and develop realistic expectations of how technology can be leveraged to overcome some of these challenges.

In Chap. 1, while depicting the background motivation for adopting digital contact tracing systems, we have talked about the natural advantages of using digital tools over the manual contact tracing processes, like faster notification and intimation, better scalability, ease of manageability, etc. However, to build a holistic perspective, we must learn the inherent complexities of the contact tracing process and re-evaluate the currently proposed digital automated solutions in light of that.

Dr. Eugenia Tognotti, in her historical review titled "Lessons from the history of Quarantine, from Plague to Influenza A" [6], has mentioned that, "Organized institutional responses to disease control began during the plague epidemic of 1347–1352." She pointed out that even in 1830 when the first wave of cholera outbreak reached European ports, the health officials used more or less the same strategies as those used at the time of plague. In cities, the sick people were forced by the authorities to move into "lazarettos" or isolation hospitals and the people who came in contact with the sick people or traveled from a place of outbreak were quarantined, which means, the contact tracing process was actively used to identify such people. During this time, in some countries, special laws were passed that curbed personal freedom of individuals and many times such laws were misused by the authorities to suppress political opposition. The widespread usage of social measures like quarantine or isolation conflicted with an individual's personal freedom and citizens' rights.

While there could be concerns on possible excesses or misuse of power by the authorities by exploiting the fear of the disease in masses, one can also justify such measures to a "reasonable" degree with the "right intent" in view of safeguarding the public health and for ensuring the safety or greater good of the citizens. Herein lies the core challenge of contact tracing (irrespective of whether manual or automated), where it has to delicately balance the two opposing requirements. This has been captured nicely in a recent article [4] by Dr. Shelly Fan where she has said that ". . . contact tracing has always teetered on the line between individual freedom and the good of the general public; the stigmatization of a viral scarlet letter versus keeping others safe; the price of health data sharing versus societal responsibility."

Let us understand the implication of the need where a DCTS needs to delicately balance the two opposite types of requirements. For example, on one hand, the system has to be prompt, accurate, and effective in alerting the general public of the risk of infection or exposure, while at the same time, it must not disclose the identity of a sick person. Additionally, in many countries, it may also allow a choice (or personal freedom) to that sick person on whether he/she is comfortable in sharing that status to the system. Similarly, the societal responsibility of minimal data sharing (e.g., the GDPR requirements in European countries) should not create a situation where it becomes tedious to carry out the usual epidemiological analysis of the contagion. Interestingly, this also means that a DCTS should be carefully architected in such a way that none of its features or strengths gets overused (e.g., anonymization of user data should not be done to such an extent that aggregate level analysis becomes infeasible). Otherwise, that feature or strength would become the biggest weakness or drawback of the system.

Now that we have touched upon the core challenges around the contact tracing process, let us explore a vision of an ideal version of the system before we settle down with a realistic one. As we go through the descriptions of these systems, it becomes apparent that, while a digital contact tracing system requires a broad-spectrum engineering focus (e.g., computing, networking, designing, usability, etc.), at the core of it lies cryptology, which is the primary motivation for us to consider a cryptologic approach for this book.

4.2 An Ideal System

In this section, we allow ourselves to indulge in imagining a system (or more appropriately, a framework of systems) that may maximize the desirability factor of users. So we request the reader to temporarily suspend the other two perspectives—feasibility and viability for the time being and focus solely on a system that can be termed "ideal" from the user's point of view.

The motivation for envisaging an ideal system comes from two fronts. First, it would give us the independence and freedom to bring innovative ideas and start the conceptualization process of digital contact tracing systems without getting constrained or influenced by the approaches already undertaken by the currently implemented (or proposed) protocols, APIs and apps. Second, it would act as a basis for us to compare a realistic framework and understand to what extent that framework may fall short of an ideal framework of the future.

The primary users of a DCTS are the individuals who at any instant of time, can be in different states of infection as per an epidemiological model, including (but not limited to)—susceptible or at risk or infected or diagnosed or recovered, etc. The secondary users would include the health authorities, the administrative authorities and the epidemiologists. There could be a third category of users who are interested to attack the system individually or as a collective, colluding group and may even attempt to influence a regular user (from the first two categories) to work in accordance with their directions temporarily or for an extended period of time. For this third category of users with malicious intent (or malicious users), the ideal system should not be desirable at all or, in other words, the system should appear to them completely unusable. We also assume that the first two categories of users always have positive intents and the only time they may behave with some negative intent (as rogue users) would be the time when they get somehow influenced by the malicious users.

Expected functionality from the perspective of primary users could be as follows.

1. The system should have the provision to track whether a user (A) came in contact, within a certain number of days in the past (as guided by the epidemiologists), either directly or through a chain of intermediate contacts, with another user (B) who has been diagnosed positive. The risk-score (signifying the probability of being infected) should factor in various epidemiological parameters including (but not limited to), how directly (or indirectly) A came in contact with B, the number of days that have elapsed since the first contact event (as well as each of the intermediate contact events for indirect contacts), the distances between every pair of individuals who directly came in contact with another person in

that chain of contacts, the duration of each of those contact events, etc. This requirement may seem mind-boggling, but it is in no way far-fetched. Imagine a situation, where A, who is infected but pre-symptomatic, happens to infect a co-traveler Asha, while commuting in the local train on her way to office. The same day, Asha transmits the virus to his office colleague Hari and from Hari after a few more hops and steps the contagion jumps and infects B by that evening. In a few days, B feels unwell, develops symptoms and tests SARS-CoV-2 positive, whereas it takes almost 21 days for A to feel sick and develop symptoms. Eventually, she also tests positive. The rest of the people in that chain may remain asymptomatic or presymptomatic for some time and suppose most of them become infectious. Shouldn't we, in this situation, expect that as soon as B tests positive, the DCTS helps us to somehow trace back to all the members in that chain of contacts starting with A? None of the currently proposed automated contact tracing systems is equipped to achieve this functionality and in the worst case may not raise a flag for the next 21 days while A, Asha and many others continue to infect other people, unknowingly, when they come in their proximity.

2. There should be negligible *false positive* or *false negative* cases. We must point out that this condition does not imply that every contact marked "at-risk" by the system is expected to be diagnosed positive (or every person declared as "not-at-risk" by the system is expected to be diagnosed negative), but rather the system should behave as closely as possible to a human contact tracer in terms of arriving at a decision, given the same set of information about a person coming in proximity to an infected person.

3. The user should be allowed to choose any app approved by an administrative authority of the person's country of residence based on his/her liking or usability preference and he/she should be free to choose a different app at any point of time. Irrespective of the app he/she chooses, a basic contact tracing service should be available to seamlessly handle the device-side or server-side contact tracing data in such a way that neither he/she should miss any critical alert (e.g., "at-risk" notification) nor the system should lose any data meant for others.

4. The system should be accessible from any type of mobile device (smartphone or feature-phone) irrespective of the model, manufacturer, or operating system, although some functionalities may be unavailable in some of those types, models, or operating systems. If a user has multiple devices, he/she should be able to designate any of those devices as the primary one for the purpose of DCTS. There must be a one-on-one correspondence between a user and his/her DCTS account.

5. There should be provision to use a basic set of functionalities of DCTS across regional, state, or national boundaries as long as the local authority participates in a federated system or at least allows access to a remote system owned by a different authority.

6. The framework should be robust against any single device or data repository failure.

7. The system should not seek any personal or personally identifiable data except any one personal data that would be securely used by the registration module to ensure that each user has a single account.

8. The personally identifiable data should be securely stored in such a way that no entity other than the registration module should be able to identify or use that; in case the registration module or database gets compromised, the system should have an in-built mechanism to either destroy the sensitive data or encrypt it in such a way that it becomes impossible to decrypt by any entity in the future.

9. The system should have the ability to mask the history of interactions in such a way that the creation of interaction graphs or social graphs becomes impossible from the available information.

10. The risk-score computation must be dynamic and reflect a recent evaluation (if not instantaneous) of the risk of infection for a user. Risk-scores should not be stored as a static value because a person who was considered *at-risk* yesterday may no longer be considered *at-risk* today.

11. The system should be intelligent enough to provide an individualized recommendation to a user based on his/her age, general health condition, travel history, etc., apart from the computed risk-score, about whether the user is *at risk* or not and if *at risk* what next step he/she should take. In this way, the system would behave like an expert human contact tracer and not share recommendations for next steps blindly. The system should also have mechanisms to learn and adapt as the system matures and as per the evolving understanding of the epidemiologists. Here, any additional data shared by the user must be handled in a secured manner without any breach of privacy.

12. Finally, the system should be useful to gauge the probability of a user of being *at-risk-of-infection* or *at-risk-of-exposure* in a way better than the random chance, even when very few users adopt or use the system.

Expected functionality from the perspective of health authorities could be as follows.

1. The system should be capable of quickly adapting to any change recommended by the health authorities with respect to the risk-scoring approach and algorithm. A more advanced system should allow the health authorities to carry out *what-if analysis* by changing one or more algorithmic parameters and thereby analyzing how that may affect the number of *at-risk* users starting from the overall system level down to small neighborhood level without revealing actual identities of any user.

2. Designated health agencies should have the sole authority to validate if a user has been *diagnosed positive* and hence whether he/she is allowed to notify the same to the system and carry out the next steps. The system should also have mechanisms using which the health authority can reverse the status to *negative* either retrospectively or from a current time onwards.

3. The health authority/designated health agencies should have authenticated communication channels through the system to communicate with the administrative authority as well as the epidemiologists.

4. Using the system, the health authority/designated health agencies should be able
   to disseminate additional guidance and advisories to the primary users to help
   them fight the pandemic situation in a better way.

Expected functionality from the perspective of administrative authorities could be as
follows.

1. The administrative authority may logically be divided into two parts—one that
   has administrative jurisdiction with respect to the users from the political and
   legal perspective and the other with the administrative rights from the automated
   system perspective. Assuming that a country may allow multiple parallel DCTS
   to function, multiple system administration authorities would have to function-
   ally roll up to the central administration which would oversee the legislative
   framework behind the system.

2. The system administrative authority should have access to manage various functionalities like

   a. Registration of the users
   b. Sharing necessary inputs and parameters to the device-side implementation
      (like the app) at the time of initialization
   c. Setting up the server-side implementation (for centralized or decentralized
      server-based systems) or distributed bulletin boards (for blockchain-based
      distributed and decentralized systems)
   d. Changing of configurable parameters including the risk-scoring algorithm
      based on recommendations from epidemiologists and/or health authority
   e. Gracefully shutting down the system at the end of the pandemic
   f. Purging of user-specific data at regular intervals based on epidemiological
      recommendations or upon explicit user request
   g. Roll out system upgrades
   h. Storage and/or dissemination of protected yet sensitive data (e.g., pseudonyms
      of users who have been diagnosed as positive, risk-scores of users in case of
      centralized risk evaluation process, etc.) in the system in a secured way
   i. Communicate with federated system administrative entities of other countries
      or regions to evaluate the risk-score of its own user in presence of users visiting
      from other countries or help the other federated system administration to
      evaluate the risk-score of that foreign user.
   j. If there happens to be a standards body in future—maintain authenticated
      communication channels with their server(s) for information exchange.

3. The system administrative authority of DCTS must have a mechanism to interface with the central administrative authority to receive common inputs from it
   (like referring to the legal obligations that a user must have based on the laws of
   the land that gets reflected in the Terms and Conditions during the registration
   process) and sharing relevant information back to the central authority for the
   purpose of reports, reviews, verification, and auditing.

Expected functionality from the perspective of epidemiological authorities could be
as follows.

1. There can be multiple epidemiological authorities who can query the system administrative authority to get aggregate level information (e.g., the number of infected users in a particular region, the density of interactions on an instantaneous and average basis, the probable hotspot regions, etc.) to track the evolution of the pandemic and measure the impact of control measures like lockdown, social distancing, quarantine, isolation, etc.
2. There should be a designated epidemiological authority (which can also be reassigned from time to time) that guides the system administrator to modify the epidemiological parameters (like how many days in the past the contact should be traced back for possible infection) and control the process of identifying at-risk users (by modifying the risk-scoring algorithms, etc.).

For the third category of users (*malicious users*), the ideal system must be robust enough to handle all possible adversarial attacks and thereby render the system completely unusable from the perspective of such malicious users with ill intent.

4.3 Attack Scenarios

An ideal system should be able to withstand all the following types of known attacks and possibly many more types of attacks that have not yet been discussed among the cryptographic community. The types of attacks can be broadly classified into the following three categories.

1. **Integrity violating attacks:** These are the attacks that mainly violate the integrity of a user's (or app's) state by introducing false positive or false negative cases, where a user's app erroneously identified the user to be *at-risk* or *not-at-risk* respectively. So far in the implementation or in the literature of automated contact tracing, higher order contact tracing (i.e., tracing close contacts of those who have come in close contact of the infected individuals) has not been considered. However, if there happens to be such a DCTS, false positive may also include cases where the app incorrectly declares the user to be at risk after coming in contact with a certain number of at-risk users (depending on the risk-scoring algorithm). In this subsection, we would outline some of the examples of false positive attack types like replay attacks, relay attacks, and Inverse-Sybil attacks, and a few examples of false negative attack types, e.g., server data breach attacks and backend impersonation attacks. Note that there could be additional types of integrity violating attacks like tampering the proximity data stored locally in devices, that have not yet been discussed in the literature because a concrete approach to accomplish any such attack has not been identified. Similarly, there could be other means of compromising a device through ransomware attack, masquerading attack, etc., that may end up showing false positives or false negatives. There is also a possibility of a device being compromised by falling in the hands of *bad actors* due to coercion threats or device misuse attack. We are not discussing any such type of attack here that may arise due to virus, malware,

bugs in the operating system, or incorrect user actions (like clicking on an unsafe link or installing a compromised app).

2. **Privacy violating attacks:** In this class of attacks, a user's personal or personally identifiable data may get leaked or compromised. Usually, a user's phone number, location, address, contact details, interaction graph, etc., fall under the category of personal or personally identifiable data. If an app collects any such data then it can be susceptible to privacy-violating attacks. Even if the app does not use any such data and work with pseudonyms or pseudorandom numbers, there could be ways to track a user by capturing additional metadata beyond the app (like video footage or snapshots) and correlating or linking such metadata with app's data for deanonymizing the user's identity. There could also be ways to mount side-channel attacks (e.g., observing when a large set of data sets get uploaded from a device to a server or identifying the time-gaps between packets transmitted between neighboring devices) that end up disclosing sensitive information about a user. A large class of offensives that violate an individual's privacy can be grouped under deanonymization attacks. Server data breach attack, device misuse attack, or coercion threats can also end up disclosing personal or personally identifiable data of a user.

3. **Usability-impacting attack:** If the usability of an app can be hampered or blocked by any attack, then that would fall under the class of usability violating attacks. A typical example of such an attack is called Denial of Service (DoS). Usability may also get severely impacted due to masquerading attacks, ransomware attacks, and deliberate injection of device or communication failures which are applicable in general for any mobile device.

Now let us discuss several attacks briefly.

Replay attack: A replay attack is a "person-in-the-middle" type of attack in which the received packets from a user's (say A's) app is captured by another user Carol who saves it in her device (through a compromised app) and later on replays the packet at a different location to B, Ted and Harry. Later, if A is found to be infected and is diagnosed positive, then the system may erroneously identify B, Ted and Harry to be at risk, although these users have never come in-proximity to any infected user.

Relay attack: A relay attack is similar to a replay attack, but it is expected to be executed in real time. That means between two devices, one or more malicious users may collaborate through a set of devices to relay the packets back and forth between the two devices at either end of that relay-chain. The effect is equivalent to that of the replay attack by introducing false positive cases in the system, however, relay attacks are inherently harder to detect and thwart as compared to replay attacks.

Inverse-Sybil attack: In this attack, a malicious user manages to use a number of devices through a single user identity. In this way, it may distribute the devices across different locations and increase the probability of coming in close proximity of an infected user. In fact, it may replicate the user-id of an actual infected user and create a large number of false positives in the system because the app running on any other device coming in proximity with the compromised devices using the same user-id as the infected user may erroneously detect contact events. This attack derives its name from the *Sybil attack*. Wikipedia says

> In a Sybil attack, the attacker subverts the reputation system of a network service by creating a large number of pseudonymous identities and uses them to gain a disproportionately large influence. It is named after the subject of the book Sybil, a case study of a woman diagnosed with dissociative identity disorder.

The Sybil attack may not have as acute an impact on DCTS as the inverse-Sybil attack. However, a large-scale version of the Sybil attack may disturb the epidemiological analysis of infection in a locality or region.

False reporting attack: If a malicious user is able to fool the system by falsely reporting diagnosed positive status while not being infected (e.g., forging the Health Authority' approval token or stealing such a token before it gets detected) or manipulating the risk computation algorithm or the risk status of an app in any other way, it would be categorized under False reporting attack. Most of the DCT Systems are expected to be robust against this type of attack.

Deanonymization attack: In this class of attack, a malicious group of users on their own or with the help of colluding authority may manage to deanonymize the identities of infected users. The approach can be based on gathering a set of information at multiple locations and then correlating those data points to deanonymize user identities or getting privileged access to private or secured datasets or utilizing some metadata information (like video footage of customers in a shopping line) beyond the DCT System. The single-entry attack is a special type of the deanonymization attack, in which a user keeps his/her device near the device of a user (without physically coming in proximity) in a vulnerable place like hospital and switching off the app otherwise. Later, if the malicious user's app declares the user at risk, then it would be easy to conclude that the original user must have been infected as the malicious user's device was never brought in close proximity to any other device intentionally. There could be various other ways to achieve deanonymization. For example, in BLE packets, the MAC address field may be used to detect whether the packets are coming from the same physical device or not. Even if the address happens to change after some time, unless that change is synchronized with the change of proximity identifier, there can always remain some chance of linkability of two packets and hence tracking users through such linking.

Server data-breach attack: A DCTS may have different types of servers (backend servers, distributed hash-tables, health authority server, bulletin board server, etc.). If any of these server's data gets breached, sensitive personal or personally identifiable user data may get leaked and/or compromised. Server data-breach may also lead to violation of the system integrity by having false positives or false negatives. In the worst case, such leakage may lead to state surveillance, blackmailing by malicious actors, or receiving threats by terrorist or militia groups.

Backend impersonation attack: In this class of attacks, the backend (which may include the registration/initialization server, contact detection server, Health Authority server, etc.) being impersonated by a fraudulent server. The effects of such an attack can be on all fronts, i.e., violation of system integrity, violation of privacy, or disruption of system usability.

Denial of Service (DoS) attack: A typical case of a DoS attack may occur at the BLE layer itself where a group of hostile devices may keep pumping in junk packets to a targeted device and thereby overwhelming the app running in that device with the processing of useless packets. Due to such processing overload, the actual contact tracing process may get hampered—hence effectively causing a denial of service. There are certain attacks applicable at the Bluetooth layer (like Bluejacking, Bluesnarfing, Bluebugging, etc.), which may end up behaving like a DoS attack. There is also a possibility of a DoS attack that affects the servers or impacts the communication channel between the device and the server(s).

Device misuse attack: If an infected user who has been diagnosed positive deliberately allows his/her device to be placed in a busy location (like a marketplace) where the app continues to share and collect proximity data packets with a large number of other devices, that device may end up generating a large number of false positives in the system which could lead to a panic situation in that locality. The infected user may also attach the device to a moving vehicle (say a vehicle that delivers essential items) or even a street dog and, in that way, the false positive cases may come up at various places and not just limited to a single locality.

Coercion attack: This is a general class of attacks where a person may come under some threat by a *bad actor* or a group of people with malicious intent who may gain access to some personal or personally identifiable data through the app or abuse the data contained in the device to cause false positives or false negatives or some other type of panic in the system. There is also a possibility of that malicious set of people blackmailing or maligning the reputation of a person using the access to such a system.

Miscellaneous types of attacks: There can be a large class of attacks that can be mounted by utilizing the possible weaknesses of the cryptographic algorithms or leakage of secret key(s) of such algorithms that are used at various stages of communication or storage of sensitive data. We do not talk about those separately in this section. We also do not explore the possibility of complex attacks that can be engineered by rebuilding the global interaction graphs or social graphs around a set of nodes defined by pseudonymous identifiers. However, an ideal system must be able to overcome any such attack that has already been discussed in the literature or may come up in due course of time.

4.4 A Realistic and Aspirational System

Why is the ideal system not a realistic one? There are quite a few reasons. First and foremost, at the lowermost level of communication, automated contact tracing systems are proposed on top of Bluetooth Low Energy (BLE) technology which was not originally designed for contact tracing purpose and hence the expectation that it could be used for that application with the desired level of accuracy and precision can be questionable. Hence, the requirement that

> The system should be accessible from any type of mobile device (smartphone or feature-phone) irrespective of the model, manufacturer or operating system.

is not realistic at this point. Similarly, the need that

> The system should be useful to gauge the probability of a user of being at-risk-of-infection or at-risk-of-exposure in a way better than the random chance, even when very few users adopt or use the system.

could be infeasible at this point as governments of almost all countries have high-lighted that the success of automated contact tracing system is singularly dependent upon the factor of how many users eventually decide to adopt and actively use the system.

In this section, we shall describe a high-level outline of a system that is both realistic and aspirational. The high-level outline will be divided into three parts—(1) an outline of a meta-framework and the need for standardization, (2) a generalized system that adheres to the meta-framework and proposed standardization, and finally, (3) an analysis of the proposed system from the cryptographic and architectural viewpoints. The reason for calling this system aspirational will be evident when we present the analysis, however, while describing a specific system we would show how the presently implemented and/or proposed solutions significantly fall short of the expectations when we compare those with the ideal system described in the previous subsection.

4.4.1 An Outline of a Meta-Framework

A meta-framework is a framework of frameworks. Here, we first describe the need for standardization from which the building blocks of the meta-framework emerge, followed by an outline of the meta-framework along with the components of standardization. Our idea is to provide a motivation and a direction rather than describe it in minute details. Moreover, one can always come up with a different variant and possibly an improved version of such a meta-framework.

4.4.1.1 Need for Standardization

Inherent non-homogeneity of any process necessitates standardization. In the absence of that standardization, the experience of users of that process suffers one way or the other. In case of contact tracing process, the inherent non-homogeneity stems from the following realities.

Coexistence of manual and digital contact tracing: In any country that has already rolled out or in the process of rolling out some digital contact tracing system, it would invariably co-exist with manual contact tracing process, simply because there are some people (e.g., children or aged members) in a family who may not be using separate devices and hence they would need to be traced manually once some other family member gets infected. Also, almost every country has an existing manual contact tracing department, its associated personnel, protocols, and procedures as part of its central health authority who might have so far used manual contact tracing in case of controlling any infectious outbreak in the past. It would be highly unlikely that they would dismantle such an existing infrastructure once DCTS is launched. Hence, the manual and digital contact tracing would co-exist. In that case, the risk computation algorithm of DCTS should be able to factor in the additional informa-tion available from manual contact tracing process. For example, a user's app may decide that the user is not at risk based on available exposure data—but when that is combined with a manual contact tracer's information of the user's exposure through another infected user's report (during interview), the combined exposure may put him/her in *at-risk* status. Similarly, there needs to be an understanding of how to resolve legal quandary. For example, if a DCTS user (say *B*) is reached out by a human contact tracer requesting him to get tested and he tests positive, would he be allowed to exercise his choice of not sharing the exposure database with the DCTS system's backend or the bulletin board (whichever may be applicable)?

Coexistence of multiple digital contact tracing systems: Surprisingly, every digi-tal contact tracing system's design documentation has so far assumed that all users in the world would have an app as per that design. Even in the specifications that have talked about federated server systems in the backend (like BlueTrace or ROBERT), the assumption is that various countries would follow the same protocol and APIs, it's only in the configurable parameters and in the app's user interface level one may come across country-specific variations. In reality, the situation is vastly different. In Europe, in spite of the formation of Pan-European Privacy-Preserving Contact Tracing body, several competing specifications and protocols have already emerged and with the advent of Apple/Google protocol, the complexity has increased further with many countries deciding in one direction and then revising their approaches. The same has recently happened in the case of the United Kingdom as well which has now announced that they would adopt the Google/Apple protocol with certain features of their existing NHS_COVID-19 app based on their experience from the initial test roll-out. In the United States, the overall variations would be even more with each state independently deciding on their adoption strategies. With the gradual removal of lockdown measures in different parts of the world and with more and more movement of people across borders, it would not be hard to imagine that soon people from different countries or even states would come in proximity to each other while running different DCTS apps on their devices which are not designed to talk to each other. If this is allowed to continue in this manner, the users would suffer big time as the apps would fail to notify them of the possible exposures. The health authorities and epidemiologists would also be unable to gauge the real-time situation of the spread of the pandemic as the aggregate data would be incomplete. In fact, it is not clear at this point in time if a country decides to switch its adoption from one DCTS system/protocol to another system/protocol what would happen to the existing data stored in users' devices or in central servers or bulletin boards (wherever they are applicable). Without standardization of how multiple DCT Systems may talk to each other the entire effort of leveraging technology may fall flat.

Differences in legal requirements: The law of the land plays an important role when it comes to an app recommending the next steps, once he/she is diagnosed positive or identified to be at-risk. If A is traveling to a new country or a region, her existing app may not be equipped to handle the new norms and regulations as per the local laws around COVID-19. In the United States, there are state-to-state variations as well. For example, in the CDC site, it is mentioned in a page [3] that "*Some states require mandatory testing for specific circumstances. Local decisions depend on local guidance and circumstances.*" Hence, there must be some mechanism in the backend among the different administrative authorities of all the DCT Systems to communicate the specific legal restrictions of each region or country and the app must be designed to reflect the local context of the user dynamically.

Additional differences: There could be additional reasons as mentioned below.

- For example, a user may have multiple DCTS apps installed in her device and, at one point of time, she may use any one of those apps. For example, if A happens to travel frequently between her country of residence (say France) and her country of work (say Germany), she may find it convenient to install both the countries' apps and use the French and German apps interchangeably as per her location dynamically, shouldn't the two apps' exposure databases have some means to communicate with each other?
- Another reason could be that there would eventually be some messaging-based systems designed for people who happen to use feature phones. The coexistence of such devices with smartphones would require the exposure information (to a positively diagnosed user of that system) to be accessible by DCTS user's app and vice versa.
- If surface transmission gets captured independently by a different type of protocol or system in the future, there must be a way for DCT Systems to utilize that information in the background.
- We need not assume that all DCT Systems would be based on BLE in future as well. If any other technology (either already present in devices like WiFi scanning or a

new technology invented later by some manufacturers) then interoperability among BLE-based DCTS and non-BLE-based DCTS would also necessitate a standardization through a meta-framework specification. It must also be noted that currently even in BLE, different protocols are using different approaches—for example, some protocols are using BLE in broadcast topology mode (like Apple/Google, DP3T, etc.), while some protocols and apps are using the connected topology mode (like BlueTrace, TraceTogether, COVIDSafe, etc.). Even in broadcast topology mode, some are using the standard 31-byte payload (like Google/Apple) while some other protocol (like ROBERT) is using the Scan Response mode as the payload there is larger than 31 bytes. During the implementation of TraceTogether in Singapore, extensive calibration has been done with respect to the signal strengths for different device manufacturers (else RSSI values may not get standardized). Such calibration and standardization would be almost imperative for every type of DCTS implementation and the country to country implementation experience may vary.

Based on all the above, we can arrive at the conclusion that it is necessary to create a meta-framework that would provide the basis for standardization of design, implementation and roll-out of DCTS systems across countries as well as their interworking with each other and with the human-led contact tracing process in the best interest of regular users, health authorities, epidemiologists, and the administrators. We have already started observing the repercussions of lack of standardization (e.g., lack of adoption of some apps due to OS-related restrictions, reversal of strategy of which protocol or system to go for, etc.) in different countries.

4.4.1.2   The Components of Standardization

This subsection is called an outline of a meta-framework because we do not intend to present a full-fledged specification here. To create such a standard, it is important to organize a forum that can interface with different design groups, private and public organizations, research institutes and bodies dedicated to automated contact tracing solutions, authorities, and administration so as to ensure that pertinent details are not missed and also to have the requisite buy-in from the various stakeholders involved. Hence, we focus on describing a high-level view of the components that should ideally be part of such a generic framework or standard.

Risk modeling: The risk modeling should primarily be guided by epidemiological considerations. The basic unit of this model can be a contact event (or exposure event). Some of the pertinent questions that the meta-framework would need to answer are listed below.

• What are the mandatory parameters that a digital contact tracing system must consider (like duration of the two parties coming in proximity to each other, the minimum average distance between them—could be measured in terms of signal strength, etc.) two determine that an *exposure* happened? Are there any other recommended or optional parameters based on which the risk modeling may depend?

- What are the risk levels to be considered (at-risk and not-at-risk or high-risk, medium-risk, low-risk, etc.) at the minimum?
- How does the risk computation depend upon the possible direct contact events (in the last 14 or 21 days or so) with those individuals who have been diagnosed positive or indirect contact events with those identified by the system as *at-risk* (secondary contacts) or even tertiary order contacts? How should the risk computation factor in information coming through human-led contact tracing process or any other means?
- Would there be an optional provision to include possible additional false positives in a probabilistic manner to counter certain types of attacks?
- Which of the above parameters should be exposed to administrators as configurable so that the risk algorithm can be tweaked post-roll-out?
- What type of details (as mentioned above) would be transparent to the regular user? What kind of aggregate information be mandatorily exposed to health authority or epidemiologists?
- How should the risk be computed—dynamically at the time of the corresponding query or at a regular interval? Would there be a scope of storing such scores—in that case at what frequency would that score get refreshed? What are the optional choices for storage of such sensitive information and what would be the security requirements?

Threat modeling: The threat modeling is a security consideration. The basic units of this model are the given trust level of entities (e.g., trusted or semi-trusted backend servers), types of malicious entities, and the mandatory attacks against which the system must be robust. Some of the issues that the meta-framework would need to consider are as follows.

- What are the types of attacks against which a digital contact tracing system must be robust? What are the types of attacks against which the system must be resilient (e.g., even if there is a compromise of server data, the system can detect and overcome such issues in a certain time-frame)? It is extremely important for a system to adhere to certain minimum standards, otherwise, we may unknowingly accept a system vulnerability. For example, the latest BLE specification [2] of Apple/Google protocol has the vulnerability of deanonymization of infected users in the same way as depicted by Vaudenay in his analysis [7] of DP3T. In the absence of any standards, we have no choice at this point other than accept the decision of the two technical giants when it comes to using the Apple/Google protocol for Exposure Notification.
- If the system detects any threat attempted against it, then what kind of log should the system maintain in order to analyze, audit, or report such events to the system administration?
- How should the system handle the knowledge of new types of threats in the future? This question could be related to the version upgrade part of the standards.

Privacy modeling: This is also a part of the security consideration. In privacy modeling, the meta-framework should answer the following types of questions—

- What type of data must be considered as personal or personally identifiable by the system?
- What type of data must not be collected by the system even in encrypted or deanonymized form? What type of data must not be collected unless encrypted or anonymized?
- What are the mandatory constraints around the storing of personal or personally identifiable data that the system must follow?
- What kind of data of a user that must not be available to another user (even in encrypted form)? What kind of data of a user that must not be made available to another user unless encrypted or anonymized?

Registration step: This is an architectural consideration. This part of the standard should indicate mandatory constraints on (a) how many accounts (or user ids or login ids) an individual is allowed to create, (b) whether the person can access his/her account(s) from multiple (or different) devices, (c) what kind of personally identifiable information (like phone number or e-mail id) the system is allowed to cross-reference at the registration step for validation, (d) whether the personally identifiable information used during the validation step can be kept (in encrypted or unencrypted fashion) for the entire life cycle of the user in the system or if it is required to be deleted, (e) if a user loses the login credentials how can he/she retrieve the same, (f) how can a user access multiple login instances (g) what kind of mandatory parameters associated with the system (e.g., number of days the exposure data can be kept in the local device storage) should be shared with the app at the time of registration (h) any mandatory cryptologic requirement etc.

Proximity data sharing: This is an architectural consideration. This part of the standard should indicate mandatory constraints on (a) packet length, (b) coding and cryptologic requirements, (c) metadata, (d) unique service identifier to differentiate one system packet with another, (f) maximum data footprint size for an event, etc.

Contact detection and exposure data sharing: These are also architectural considerations. This part of the standard should indicate mandatory constraints on (a) max time-limit within which the contact detection must happen after an infected user (who earlier came in proximity to the current user) is known to be positive, (b) validity or time-limit of authorization token given by health authority in case of data upload, (c) coding and cryptologic requirements, (d) maximum data footprint for the related events, etc.

De-registration: This is an architectural consideration. This part of the standard should indicate mandatory constraints on (a) data cleanup and data retention process (connected with legal requirements as well), (b) reuse of login id by any other user in future, (c) inclusion of required information (about the data) for aggregate computation purposes (to be later on referred by epidemiologists), etc.

Fault modeling: This is also an architectural consideration which should outline the mandatory requirements for system resilience against different types of failures and data losses. Incidentally, none of the currently proposed protocols and systems has talked about this aspect.

Additional areas: There are various other areas around which standardization would be required like (a) communication among backend servers (like system administrative server and health authority server), (b) communication among federated servers of the same protocol or system or between two different systems, etc.

   The components of standardization can also be viewed in terms of network layers, like the following

1. **Physical and link layer:** The physical and link layer communication meta-framework involves the descriptions and usage of different physical layer technologies (BLE, Bluetooth, WiFi, etc.), the constraints of their usage and the definition of the hardware abstraction layer to create a standardized approach so that the higher layers may send/receive the packets in a way that is independent of the actual technologies being used.

2. **Network layer:** This is the main API layer that is used by the app which eventually gets translated in the form of link layer APIs that abstract the hardware interface. Since the hardware abstraction layer is not expected to impose any particular type of encryption/decryption or encoding/decoding algorithm, that critical functionality must be handled by the network layer APIs. So in a way, for any DCTS, this layer forms the heart of the security and privacy architecture and hence the meta-framework needs to define certain standard approaches that must be adhered to by all the DCT Systems in this layer.

3. **App layer:**

   a. **User interface part:** User interface part describes the way a user can make use of the contact tracing system, what other functionalities would be available to the user apart from the contact tracing and how the configurable parameters would be exposed by the system that requires user intervention and/or approval.

   b. **Client-server communication part:** This part is usually not transparent to the user. But important characteristics of the system in each phase of registration, initialization, de-registration, status notification, exposure detection, etc., can be standardized through this layer.

   c. **Server-to-server communication part:** A large-scale protocol standardization is required for defining the process in which heterogeneous systems can inter-operate across geographic or regional boundaries.

Any standard should also indicate optional as well as recommended parts. There could also be areas included as "must-not," e.g., the standard may prevent the apps to include any other notifications that go beyond contact tracing requirements and may be viewed as either propaganda or commercial advertisements.

4.5 A High-Level Description of a Generalized System

In this section, we provide a high-level description of a generalized system that would meet some of the expectations of an ideal system, which are not yet available in any of the designs described in Chaps. 2 and 3 under Centralized and Decentralized varieties. To maintain the brevity of the book's structure, we describe an outline of the system and not a detailed design specification. Also, we assume that eventually there would be a standard meta-framework available which all DCT systems in the world would adhere to and hence our proposed system would be able to exploit certain features of that meta-framework. In absence of any such standard (or meta-framework), certain aspects of this proposed system would not be realizable or practically implementable. Since in this section, our intent is to offer a more generalized approach as compared to any special purpose architecture, let us call the proposed system, a Generalized Digital Contact Tracing System (GDCTS) or *System-G* in short that utilizes a meta-framework referred to as *Framework-M*.

We start describing System-G from a network layer perspective.

Physical and link layer communication: Assuming that the *Framework-M* would take care of the link layer protocol, *System-G* should not be dependent on a specific hardware interface (like BLE). The *Framework-M* would provide the required abstraction to hide the physical implementation details and expose a standard set of link layer APIs to the higher level layer (network layer). The *Framework-M* would be expected to be used by every other DCTS in the world so that the benefit of hardware layer abstraction is available to other systems as well. *System-G* would additionally exploit the link layer uniformity by implementing the system in such a way that the data packets from any other device in proximity, running some other automated contact tracing protocol that adheres to *Framework-M*, can be utilized and factored in to identify the risk of infection. In absence of a deployed *Framework-M*, the proposed *System-G* would be able to work only in a homogeneous environment (i.e., allow communication between devices that are running *System-G*-based apps only) and not in a heterogeneous environment where it may analyze packets coming from any DCTS app.

In the absence of any meta-framework and assuming that the physical implementation would utilize the BLE interface, *System-G* would have to define its own data link layer protocol. In case there exists a deployment of a meta-framework, the definition of the physical layer packets (using BLE technology) could also adhere to the following guideline.

- BLE interface would use the *Broadcast* topology and the packet size would be limited to the standard 31 bytes—hence there would not be a need to use the *Scan-*

Response mode. The primary intent behind this guideline is to keep the device to device communication light-weight. Moreover, by avoiding the *Connected* topology or *Scan-Response* mode in the *Broadcast* topology, one may expect to achieve higher throughput.

- Each packet will contain 2–4 bytes of Encrypted Metadata (EM) apart from the pseudonymous pseudo-andom ID (12–16 bytes) to store information like signal strength and a byte of information to indicate the maximum number of days the packet may be retained in the device. The service data part of the payload should also include a Message Authentication Code (MAC) so that data tampering can be detected. The idea is inspired in the way ROBERT protocol has incorporated MAC in its HELLO packet. However, we are not specifying the exact algorithm to be used for generating the MAC or proposing any specific length at this stage because the detailed design specification will eventually depend upon *Framework-M* as well.
- The advertisement and gathering of proximity data packets will happen transparently in the background. Currently, in Apple devices, no app is allowed access to BLE in the background mode. Therefore, it would be desirable that Apple and Google either come up with a meta-framework or align with the efforts that may be undertaken by a standards body to define a *Framework-M*. In absence of such an implementation from Apple/Google, System-G would have to abide by the current OS-specific constraints, which means that the app may not properly function unless it runs in the foreground. It must be pointed out that in almost all the mobile devices there is a provision to separately keep *Bluetooth scanning* mode ON even when Bluetooth is switched OFF. This is the configuration in which apps can continue to run in the background provided the OS layer supports the access to the BLE.
- The packet should have two separate indicators (a) a UUID value to signify the class of service (e.g., 0xFD6F can be used in line with Apple/Google's for Exposure Notification Service ID) and (b) a sub-service SSID (included in the service data part), to indicate the exact protocol (this can be defined by some standards).
- There should be a provision in the implementation to store the packets in such a way that any DCTS app installed in the device can access the packets. Essentially, this is the concept of creating an abstraction layer through a meta-framework so that the storage of packets gets independently handled by a common proximity data access service. Of course, the packets of one DCTS system would not be decipherable by a different app, but the interoperability architecture will still ensure that such data can be used to measure the risk-score of the user. The proximity data access service should take care of deleting the old data from the local storage, based on information contained in the packet or a default number of days (say 21 days). Incidentally, this data store will be different from the app-specific data storage where the proximity data and meta-data would be stored after necessary decoding but the database will be encrypted so that no other app can decipher these information. The common data store will serve more or less as the backup for the app-specific data—even in the situation where the app may crash and the data becomes corrupt, the common store can be referred to retrieve past data when the app gets re-installed.

Network layer: This layer would consist of the APIs that would be directly used by the app to accomplish various functions like registration, initialization, creation, and communication of proximity data after applying the encoding and encryption steps, receipt, and retrieval of the proximity data from other devices after decrypting, decoding and safely storing those in the app-specific encrypted data store, uploading of proximity data for *infected* user or at-risk user (after validation by the Health Authority), checking the bulletin board or distributed hash-table to identify the risk of coming in contact with an infected user or even an *at-risk* user, requesting the restoration of status from *infected*, or *at-risk* to *not-at-risk* status (upon validation by Health Authority) and deregistration of user. These functions in the context of System-S are described in detail later in the next few subsections.

App layer: As indicated in the description of meta-framework, the app layer specification should be divided into three parts-

1. User interface part: The UI of the System-S would provide both diagnostic guidance based as well as proximity-based risk notification to the user. The diagnosis-based risk assessment can be done through a series of questions posed to the user (it is possible to envisage that there can be an on-device AI engine that would learn from the epidemiological server the current disease transmission parameters and refine the diagnostic algorithm accordingly). In terms of contact tracing functionality, the UI should have provision to explicitly check with the user about his/her preference on

   a. Whether higher order contact tracing would be enabled (this is explained in the functionality wise description of *System-S* below)
   b. Whether to upload the proximity data in case of *infected* or *at-risk* status
   c. The choice of deregistration and withdrawal of participation at any point of time
   d. The choice of retrieval of backed-up proximity data in the device at the time of reinstalling the app (for some reason)
   e. The choice of participating in the federated interoperable DCT Systems.

2. Client-server communication part: There would be three types of servers with which *System-S* may need to communicate, namely

   a. The central server that would be accessed by the app (client) only when it needs to resolve the risk status for the owner of the packets that are emitted by a different DCT System
   b. The distributed hash-table based or the bulletin board servers (possibly using blockchains) which help the apps to resolve the risk status by peer-to-peer communication via the intermediate server (this part is entirely meant for the packets belonging to *System-S*-based apps)
   c. The server belonging to the designated Health Authority which provides validation of status change (between *not-at-risk*, *at-risk*, and *infected states*).

3. Server-to-server communication part: There could be four types of server-to-server communication, as follows

    a. Federated server to server communication (from the Central server to other Central servers) to handle the movement of users across multiple states or countries (including diverse protocol-based systems)

    b. Central server to bulletin board (or distributed hash-table-based) servers) to resolve incoming query from other DCT Systems for risk status of the owner of a packet

    c. Communication of epidemiological data points between the bulletin boards (or distributed hash-tables) to the epidemiological database server (can also be a part of the Health Authority server)

    d. Communication of configuration parameters between the central administrative server and other servers/bulletin board (or distributed hash-table).

We now describe *System-S* in terms of the functional modules.

Registration: The registration process would ensure that (a) there is a proof-of-work check so that automated bots cannot create accounts, (b) each mobile device can have only one System-S user at any point of time (all past data stored in the device will automatically be deemed to belong to this user unless he/she explicitly raises a purge request, which would need additional validation steps), (c) the phone number is initially shared with the registration/admin server for validation that the user possesses the SIM card, however once a permanent user id is created at the back end with a mapping between login id of the user and the permanent id, the phone number is no longer stored and the local common storage will be created for the first time with that validation, (d) a person can access his/her account only from one device; from any other device the only option would be to create a new login id, (e) no personally identifiable information would be stored except the PIN/ZIP or equivalent code of the user that would be used later for epidemiological purposes, (f) if a user loses the login credentials he would have to create a new login id—however, the past device data and the corresponding user ids would automatically get associated with the same user, (g) a user can simultaneously access the system through multiple login ids provided he/she uses a different mobile device for each login.

Initialization: The registration step is immediately followed by the initialization step where the app received the configurable parameters from the server, approved URLs of the Health Authority's server, bulletin board (or distributed hash-table) addresses, epidemiological server, etc., and also the relevant keys that would be used to have secure and authenticated communication between the entities.

De-registration: At the time of deregistration the device-specific local data would be purged and the mapping of login id with the permanent user id at the backend server will be deleted (hence the same login id can be reused later). The proximity data records stored in the bulletin board (or in the distributed hash-table) would not be touched as it would be impossible for the server to identify which records belong to this user. Those entries will automatically get purged after the epidemiologically significant time-window is crossed.

Risk computation: This would primarily depend upon the number of close contacts (or exposures) in the past ESDays (Epidemiologically Significant Days) with either infected or *at-risk* contacts.

- The duration of the two parties coming in proximity to each other should be 10 min or more and the average distance between them (measured through calibrated RSSI parameters) should be less than 2 m.
- The risk levels would be *at-risk* and *not-at-risk*
- The risk computation algorithm will run locally and it will depend upon the possible direct contact events (in the last ESDays) detected by the bulletin board service (or distributed hash-table service) with those individuals who have been diagnosed *positive* or identified by the system as *at-risk* (secondary contacts). The actual algorithm would be downloaded by the app from the admin server once a week.
- There would not be any false positive deliberately introduced through probabilistic algorithms.
- The details of the number of contacts and types of contacts would be transparently available to the user and he/she may have an option to explicitly consult a health service professional or human contact tracer who would provide an independent evaluation of the user's risk-status. In this evaluation, the health professional can factor in additional information like age of the person, past travel history, general health condition, etc. In fact, there can also be a possibility to expose an expert system-based interface to user, where he/she may play around different parameters and find out the way risk computation varies without disclosing any sensitive personal data.
- The risk would always be computed dynamically and this information would not be stored.

Proximity data sharing between two *System-S* apps: In *System-S*, we propose a symmetric approach of proximity data sharing between two apps running *System-S* protocols. It is inspired by the DESIRE protocol where an app comes up with a secret pseudorandom number in every epoch and shares a mathematical transformation of that secret number in the form of a rolling proximity number while broadcasting to nearby devices. When another *System-S* app running in a nearby device receives that number, it applies another mathematical function based on its secret number for that epoch and saves the Transformed Proximity Number (TPN). On the other hand, when the first app receives the rolling proximity number of that epoch from the latter device, it applies the same mathematical function before saving it locally. The functions are designed in such a way that these two saved numbers can be easily matched by an independent server or a distributed server (or a distributed hash-table) even though the secret keys are not shared by any of the devices. Before saving a TPN in the app-specific database, the corresponding metadata is decrypted and from the calibrated signal strength information (which should be part of the metadata), the approximate distance between the two devices is calculated. If the distance is more than 2 m, the packet is silently dropped without saving. If the distance is acceptable, the TPN information is stored along with the decrypted metadata. If the same rolling proximity number is received by the app within one epoch (of duration 10 min) for at least 5 min, a corresponding flag is enabled in the data store to indicate that this encounter is epidemiologically significant.

The reason for keeping these two time-windows different and one with a value of 10 min, while the other with a value of 5 min, is to take into consideration that the epoch boundaries of the two apps may not be identical. If we consider that the 10 min of association of two individuals with an average distance at most 2 m is epidemiologically significant, there is a possibility of rolling proximity number of one app changing once during the 10 min epoch of the other. However, even with that change, there must be one time-window that is of the duration of at least 5 min. There is also a downside to this decision, as there could be some cases falsely reported as positive where one user may actually not stay for 10 min and still the system would flag the encounter as significant if the duration of association is around 5 min of more.

Proximity data sharing between a *System-S* app and a different DCTS app: If a *System-S* app receives a packet from a different DCTS app, it will not be able to decode that packet and hence it will simply store it within the local app-specific storage with additional metadata like the time of reception of that packet. Assuming that the received packet follows the SUID convention, it would be possible to identify the corresponding country/protocol combination that is represented by that SUID. Please note that here we are assuming a convention that the country identification is subsumed in SUID instead of following a convention of ROBERT in which the HELLO packet contains an Encrypted Country Code (ECC) separately. If a packet is present in the app-specific data store for more than *ESDays*, it would get deleted (by following a process similar to the one followed in device-specific common data-store).

4.5.1   Higher Order Contact Tracing

This is the functionality that is not present in any of the implemented or proposed systems that we have talked about in the previous two chapters. To the best of our knowledge, we have not come across such a proposal in the literature, so far. Through this functionality, a user can identify whether he/she has come in contact with some other user who has been identified in the system to be *at-risk* (and has not been diagnosed positive yet) in the past *ESDays*. We have described one such use-case while describing an ideal system. The motivation comes from the key observation of the epidemiological community across the world that apparent asymptomatic or pre-symptomatic people can also be infectious and it is important to contain the spread of the disease early enough by tracking such cases through extensive testing in the population or by launching aggressive contact tracing. If we consider a mathematical graph-like structure where each app acts as a node/vertex and we draw an edge between two nodes/vertices whenever two devices corresponding to two nodes/vertices come near each other for an epidemiologically significant duration. In that case, one can envisage the set of nodes that are reachable by a direct edge from one node as that node's immediate neighborhood. In that case, the problem of identifying the apps that have come in proximity of at-risk user apps is the same as identifying the neighborhood or neighborhood from a user's node who has been diagnosed as positive. Theoretically, this can be extended indefinitely within the same mathematical framework, but in reality, we may not need to check beyond the set of users who might have come in second-degree contact with an *infected* user. This is the functionality that we refer to in this section as *higher order contact tracing*.

Infection notification: If a user is diagnosed positive, he/she gets a token in the form of a code (like a QR code) from a Health Authority (this part of beyond *System-S*). The token permanently changes the state of the app to *InfectedUserAppStatus*. This status can be reversed only after another diagnosis where the user is declared uninfected by the Health Authority (HA) and subsequently the user receives another token from HA to restore the app's status to *UninfectedUserAppStatus* which is the initial state of an app at the time of installation. Whenever the HA releases a valid token, it keeps track of the zip/postal code of the infected user—this data is used by the epidemiologists to understand region wise infection count and disease dynamics. As soon as an app is assigned the state *InfectedUserAppStatus*, the user is asked if he/she would like to help others by uploading the proximity data received from other devices in a secured manner to the bulletin board server (or the distributed hash-table, etc.) so that other apps can check whether they came in proximity of the current app's device in the past *ESDays*. If the user gives a go ahead all the relevant data gets uploaded after getting a blind signature from the Health Authority server to the bulletin board server. In addition, the user may agree that the app would continue to upload the additional daily received data till the point it changes state to *UninfectedUserAppStatus*.

At-risk notification: Whenever the user's app determines (with the help of the bulletin board server) that a user is *at-risk*, the user would face another choice of whether he/she would like to upload the received list of proximity data to the bulletin board server so that other users can determine the events where they came in contact with at-risk users in the past *ESDays*.

It must be mentioned here that either during infection notification or during at-risk notification, the proximity data packets received from a different DCTS app are not uploaded. The processing of such packets is solely handled in the exposure detection stage as mentioned below.

Exposure detection (homogeneous case): At the exposure detection stage (in a homogeneous *System-S* app environment), each app uploads its received packets (for the past *ESDays*) once every day to the bulletin board server's exposure matching detection service which not only detects the number of contacts with *infected* individuals but also the number of exposures with at-risk users. The consolidated data counts are shared with the app where the risk-scoring algorithm determines the user's risk after factoring in additional data points that may be present only locally at the user end and not stored anywhere else due to privacy consideration. The actual matching process is similar to that of DESIRE protocol and hence we are not going into the details any further.

Exposure detection (heterogeneous case): This is possibly the most complex and advanced functionality of System-S. However, it cannot work on its own in a stand-alone fashion unless there is a federated heterogeneous server to server communication infrastructure available through *Framework-M*. In the absence of such a support meta-framework or standardized server-to-server communication among multiple DCT Systems, the packets received from other DCT Systems would have to be silently dropped and ignored. If there is an interoperable system infrastructure supported by *Framework-M*, the following can be one way to handle exposure detection in heterogeneous systems

- The app will use the bulletin board or distributed hash-table server as a post-box to keep the list of packets received within last ESDays grouped according to SUID or country/protocol system names. The backend admin server will not know the app's identity who is keeping the records. It would contact the admin or backend server of the other DCT System and resolve the question of whether any of these packets came from an infected user or not (belonging to that DCT System) and if true whether the duration of contacts was epidemiologically significant.
- Please note that for such packets, second-degree exposure detection may not be feasible as the server of that DCT System may not be maintaining such a list either centrally or in a distributed database
- If the other system is a centralized one (like BlueTrace), it could be easier to provide the required data back to the System-S admin server.
- If the received packet came from a purely decentralized DCTS, where the proximity matching service is transparently handled without the direct involvement of the admin-server, a special proxy service may need to be created at the server end to enable this kind of interoperability between heterogeneous DCT Systems.

4.6   Analysis of the Generalized System

We now present a high-level analysis of the system. First, we analyze it from the security and privacy standpoint and then carry out an architectural analysis.

4.6.1   Security Analysis

Replay attack: *System-G* can not be subjected to Replay attacks because it is designed as a system that validates a match by symmetric exchange of packets (like DESIRE protocol).

Relay attack: It should be possible to execute a Relay attack on the system as inherently no location-specific metadata has been included in the proximity data packets. However, the restriction that a contact event will be considered valid only when the packets are exchanged at least for 10 min continuously between the two targeted devices, makes the adversary's job complex. This is apart from the difficulty imposed by the symmetric nature of the protocol where the intervening set of devices have to relay the packets on both the directions to ensure that the contact event gets registered on both the devices.

Inverse-Sybil attack: Since the app can not be accessed with the same user-id from multiple devices, it would not be possible to subject *System-G* to Inverse-Sybil attack.

False reporting: We have not explicitly mentioned how the Health Authority may approve and validate the *diagnosed-positive* cases. Whenever the specific implementation of this generalized system defines the way the token would get generated, susceptibility of the system can be analyzed. One important characteristic of the *System-G* is that it also takes care of a user's state restoration as and when the user is declared diagnosed negative. Hence, the possibility of a user indefinitely remaining in the system with *infected* status is no longer feasible.

Deanonymization attack: The proximity identifiers of an infected person is not made public in this system and the matching happens transparently at the backend/bulletin-board/hash-table-based server. Hence, infected user re-identification is not possible in *System-G*. It can still be possible through other means (like the reaction of a user on coming to know of the diagnostic test result or someone overhearing a conversation of a user with a health service professional), but that does not provide the malicious user with any additional advantage as any captured proximity identifier can not be replayed later to any other user to cause confusion and panic. Single-user attack can be prevented by incorporating a risk algorithm that does not give any indication of risk to the user unless at least two direct or indirect contacts with infected status get detected.

Server data-breach attack: No personal or personally identifiable information is collected and stored in the backend. Even the bulletin board data can not be deciphered without the help of respective apps' secret keys. Hence System-G is not susceptible to the regular type of server data-breach attacks. However, in a heterogeneous system, the server to server data communication, if leaked, may reveal some information about the infected users.

Backend impersonation attack: Since we consider all the servers to use well-known domain names with the highest possible grade of security and authentication through valid certificates, this type of attack is not applicable on *System-G*.

Denial of Service (DoS) attack: There is nothing in System-G that can inherently prevent a typical DoS attack. In a specific implementation, we recommend that some deep learning-based solution should be added that must be first trained to identify junk BLE packets and then detect their presence whenever such attacks are mounted against the system.

Device misuse attack: System-G is definitely susceptible to such an attack. To prevent such an attack, there must be a mechanism (beyond DCTS) or a process to enable location congruity tracking based on the user's self-declaration.

Coercion attack: Like Device misuse attack, Coercion attack is also feasible. Hence, in that way, *false positives* may get created in the system easily. However, there is not much risk of losing personal or personally identifiable data as even the user of the app can never decipher any sensitive information on his/her own.

Social graph: The backend server/bulletin board server would not be able to create the social graph as the proximity identifiers uploaded by a user once diagnosed as positive vis-a-vis by the same app for checking its exposure are not the same and hence can not be used to construct a social graph.

4.6.2 Architecture Analysis

Extent of decentralization: The specification is given in such a way that the system can be customized to the extent required to either a fully decentralized system or somewhere in between centralized and decentralized systems.

Fault tolerance: The system can withstand single-point failure at the device end where a common data store is created that remains separate from the app-specific data store. The distributed hash-tables or bulletin board servers can also be created in the cloud to have in-built fault tolerance against any single database failure.

Interoperability: The usage of Framework-M in System-G mainly serves the purpose of interoperability in a heterogeneous environment with multiple countries or regions/states.

High-order contact tracing: This is a novel introduction which has not been proposed in any other system so far to the best of our knowledge.

Risk-computation algorithm: This has been designed in a flexible yet comprehensive way so that the final recommendation of *at-risk or not-at-risk* status can be as individualized as possible without sacrificing the privacy requirements of the system.

The expectations of an ideal system from health authority, epidemiological authority, and administrative authorities can not be studied or analyzed at this point for *System-G* as specific implementation details would be required to guide the way these authorities may access the exposed APIs of a system.

4.7 Conclusion

Writing a book on digital contact tracing systems in the midst of a life-changing pandemic feels like designing a flight-simulator for engines that have just begun their maiden voyages in turbulent weather. We do not claim that we know the final answer on what would eventually work. Therefore, as authors, we view this book as an earnest attempt to take a holistic view of this important topic with a specialized lens of cryptology. It is altogether possible that the terrain of automated contact tracing solutions would look much different after a few months and, in such a case, the later editions of the book would incorporate such changes. However, if one has to take a look at a snapshot in the time of how a set of system requirements, definitions, and designs on this important class of problem are emerging, then this book can be a reasonably good start. Moreover, in this book, we have tried to look at the problem from a medium to a long-term time-frame and hence the big picture view has enabled us to generalize certain solutions and point out the possible directions of the journey by taking into consideration the interests of multiple stakeholders, including—administrators, health authorities, epidemiologists, designers, technologists, and finally and, most importantly, the end users.

References

1. Andrew, Ng. Why AI is the new electricity? Retrieved March 11, 2017. https://www.gsb.stanford.edu/insights/andrew-ng-why-ai-new-electricity.
2. Apple and Google. Exposure notification – Bluetooth specification, v1.2, April 2020. https://covid19-static.cdn-apple.com/applications/covid19/current/static/contact-tracing/pdf/ExposureNotification-BluetoothSpecificationv1.2.pdf.
3. Centres for Disease Control and Prevention. Contact tracing for COVID-19. https://www.cdc.gov/coronavirus/2019-ncov/php/contact-tracing/contact-tracing-plan/contact-tracing.html.
4. Fan, S. Contact tracing is the next step in the COVID-19 Battle – But how will it work in western countries? Retrieved April 21, 2020, https://singularityhub.com/2020/04/21/why-bringing-contact-tracing-into-our-digital-world-is-hard-and-why-we-must-do-it-anyway/.
5. Kurzweil, R. The singularity is near. Penguin USA, 2006. https://www.amazon.in/Singularity-Near-Humans-Transcend-Biology/dp/0143037889.
6. Tognotti, E. (2013). Lessons from the history of quarantine, from plague to influenza A. *Emerging Infectious Diseases*, *19*(2), 254–259. https://www.ncbi.nlm.nih.gov/pmc/articles/PMC3559034/.
7. Vaudenay, S. Analysis of DP-3T between scylla and charybdis. Cryptology ePrint Archive, Report 2020/399. https://eprint.iacr.org/2020/399.pdf.

Index

Printed in the United States
by Baker & Taylor Publisher Services